OXFORD MEDICAL PUBLICATIONS

Cognitive Assessment
for Clinicians

D1085769

Cognitive Assessment for Clinicians

JOHN R. HODGES

University Lecturer, University of Cambridge Clinical School;
Honorary Consultant Neurologist, Addenbrooke's Hospital,
Cambridge

Oxford   New York   Tokyo
OXFORD UNIVERSITY PRESS

Oxford University Press, Great Clarendon Street, Oxford OX2 6DP

Oxford New York
Athens Auckland Bangkok Bogota Bombay Buenos Aires
Calcutta   Cape Town Dar es Salaam Delhi Florence Hong Kong
Istanbul   Karachi Kuala Lumpur Madras Madrid Melbourne
Mexico City Nairobi Paris Singapore Taipei Tokyo Toronto Warsaw
and associated companies in
Berlin Ibadan

Oxford is a trade mark of Oxford University Press

Published in the United States by
Oxford University Press Inc., New York

© John R. Hodges, 1994

First published 1994
Reprinted 1994, 1995 (with corrections), 1996, 1998

A catalogue record for this book is available from the British Library

Library of Congress Cataloging in Publication Data
(Data available on request)
ISBN 0 19 262394 X

Printed in Great Britain on acid-free paper by
Biddles Ltd, Guildford and King's Lynn

Preface

This book grew out of my experience over the past few years of teaching trainee physicians, psychiatrists, and psychologists about cognitive function and its assessment. I had initially intended to write a very brief pocket guide dealing only with bedside testing. But it became apparent that there was little value in merely describing how to assess cognition, unless the reader had some conceptual knowledge about normal psychological function on which to base the assessment and, most importantly, to guide the interpretation of the examination's findings. The book, therefore, expanded in scope and in size. It now attempts to provide a rational and theoretical basis for cognitive assessment at the bedside or in the clinic, as well as practical guidance on how to take an appropriate history and how to examine patients presenting with disorders of higher cerebral function. The approach advocated in the book is illustrated by twelve case histories of patients seen by me over the last two years. The final section consists of an appendix describing commonly used neuropsychological tests.

When writing the theoretical sections which underpin the assessment, I have drawn on two major strands of research—the traditional localizationalist approach, and the more recent cognitive neuropsychological approach. Most clinicians will be aware of the former; ever since the original observations of Broca, Wernicke, Pick, Dejerine, and others in the last century, neurologists have been interested in the cerebral localization of higher mental functions. After a period of relative neglect, recent advances in static (CT and MRI) and functional (PET and SPECT) neuro-imaging have reactivated this traditional approach, and considerable advances have been made in the localization of various cognitive functions, which I have attempted to summarize.

The other major strand, cognitive neuropsychology, will be less familiar to clinicians. Most medical curricula still contain only a rudimentary grounding in psychology, and virtually no cognitive neuropsychology. Even some psychology graduates have little experience of this area. Yet in the past two decades there has been an explosion of interest in this field which has produced unparalleled insights into the workings of the human mind. Much of this research originated in Britain, beginning with the pioneering work of John Marshall and Freda Newcombe, and of Elizabeth Warrington and her colleagues. Their experimentally based approach to dissecting the individual subprocesses underlying functions such as reading, object recognition, etc., paved the way for working out the detailed cognitive models that now exist and can be tested experimentally. These and kindred researchers have stressed the critical importance of single-case studies, and of designing tests which isolate specific and dissociable cognitive processes. I have attempted to introduce readers to this exciting area, and to provide a review of the clinically important advances that have been made in cognitive neuropsychology.

Unfortunately, the two major research traditions have, until recently, carried on independently, so that although we now know a great deal about the cognitive basis of many aspects of language, memory, and perception, the neural bases of these processes remain largely unknown. This creates problems when trying to unite these disparate approaches to neuropsychology. In places, the marriage that I have imposed between neurology and cognitive neuropsychology appears rather shaky. It is to be hoped that further advances in the next few years will consolidate our understanding in these areas.

The structure of the book is as follows. Chapters 1 and 2 deal with the theoretical aspects of cognitive function, divided into those which have a widely distributed neural basis (attention/concentration, memory, and highest-order 'executive' function), and those functions which are lateralized to one hemisphere, and often one region of one hemisphere (language, praxis, visuo-spatial and perceptual abilities, etc.). Each section of these chapters deals with the neuropsychology, the basic applied anatomy, the clinical disorders, and appropriate tests. The tests mentioned are described in more detail in the Appendix. At the end of Chapter 1 there is also a brief section on delirium and dementia, which constitute the commonest presenting disorders in behavioural neurology and old age psychiatry.

Chapter 3 describes how to take a cognitive history, with a few tips on physical examination. Chapter 4 outlines my approach to assessment at the bedside or in the clinic, and follows the same format as the earlier introductory theoretical chapters. Chapter 5 contains twelve case histories, most of which are taken from our joint neurology–psychiatry cognitive disorders clinic and illustrate the approach advocated in the earlier chapters. In Chapter 6, I describe the standardized mental test batteries in common use (for example the Mini Mental State Examination, the Blessed Informa-tion–Memory–Concentration IMC Test, the Hodkinson Brief Mental Test, the Dementia Rating Scale, and the Cambridge Cognitive Examination CAMCOG) with notes on their use and abuse. Finally, the Appendix contains details on a selection of neuropsychological tests, consisting of those widely used in neuropsychological practice, with which clinicians should be familiar, and tests which can be given fairly readily by clinicians without specialist training.

I should point out that this is not intended to be a textbook of neuropsychology, of which there are several excellent examples listed under 'Selected Further Reading' at the end of the book. Neither is it a compendium of neuropsychological tests. It is aimed at clinicians with a nascent, but underdeveloped, interest in cognitive function. The approach advocated forms no substitute for professional psychological evaluation. However, many neurologists and psychiatrists work without adequate neuropsychological provision. By becoming more conversant with bedside cognitive testing, clinicians should be able to use the services of their neuropsychologists more effectively. It is not necessary, for instance, to refer every patient with suspected dementia; many patients can be satisfactorily diagnosed by clinicians if the basic principles outlined in the book are followed. There are, however, patients in whom a thorough neuropsychological evaluation is mandatory, as is illustrated by several of the cases in Chapter 5.

If this book stimulates any trainee neurologist or psychiatrist to develop a special interest in neuropsychology, or to pursue a research career in this field, then it will have more than fulfilled its original aims.

Acknowledgements

I would like first, and foremost, to acknowledge the intellectual debt I owe to a number of teachers and colleagues who have encouraged my interest in cognitive dysfunction over the years. Whilst in Oxford, I was fortunate to work with John and Susan Oxbury, who provided an environment in which an interest in neuropsychology was encouraged. The presence of John Marshall and Freda Newcombe in the University Department of Neurology was also a seminal influence. This milieu, which was sadly unique in British neurology, also nurtured the interests of my friends and contemporaries Christopher Ward and Harvey Sagar. At that time I also began a fruitful collaboration with Elaine Funnell, who was working at Birkbeck College. Charles Warlow did much to help by co-supervising my MD project on transient global amnesia when he was Clinical Reader in Oxford, and by implanting the idea of this book on a subsequent visit to Edinburgh.

The Medical Research Council kindly sponsored a fellowship year spent studying neuropsychology at the Alzheimer Disease Research Center in the University of California, San Diego. Whilst I was there, Nelson Butters and David Salmon were particularly influential. It was this year, more than any other, that decided the direction of my future research interests.

Since moving to Cambridge, I have been extremely fortunate to work closely with a group of outstanding clinical and experimental neuropsychologists. Karalyn Patterson has been a particularly important guiding light, and together we have established an active research programme investigating aspects of language and memory in patients with Alzheimer's disease and progressive aphasia. Our research assistants Naida Graham, Elaine Hoffner, and Hilary Baddeley have allowed us the luxury of time to actually think about our research and for me to write this book. I have also benefited enormously from collaborations with Roz McCarthy, Trevor Robbins, Barbara Sahakian, Felicia Huppert, and Barbara Wilson. The other members of the neuropsychiatry research group—German Berrios, Paul Calloway, Tom Denning, Nigel Hymas, and Peter McKenna—continue to provide intellectual stimulation and support. Sections of the book were read for me by Judith Allanson, Leo Blomert, Kristin Breen, Tom Denning, Mark Doran, Jon Evans, Eleanor Feldman, Paula McKay, Karalyn Patterson, Ian Robertson, Andrew Tarbuck, and Barbara Wilson, all of whom made valuable comments. My wife, Carol Gregory, deserves special mention as the only other person to have read the entire manuscript twice. Any errors remain, however, my own doing. Illustrations of neglect patients' drawings were kindly given to me by Peter Halligan of the Rivermead Rehabilitation Hospital, Oxford. My secretary Linda Pallister tolerated many redraftings of the text.

Cambridge   J. R. H.
June 1993

To Adam and Will

Contents

1. *Distributed cognitive functions*

A general theoretical framework

When approaching cognitive assessment it is essential to have a general structure on which to base the clinical interview and examination. The schema suggested here attempts to link anatomy and cognitive function. However, the strict localization of many cognitive functions is still far from clear. In a quest for clarity and brevity, I have been forced to take a simplified and often didactic approach that necessarily avoids many interesting issues and controversies in neuropsychology. For those wishing to read more detailed analyses of structural–functional relationships, and of cognitive neuropsychology, several reference sources are suggested at the end of the book.

The basic dichotomy offered here is between distributed and localized functions. The label *distributed* implies cognitive functions which are *not* strictly localized to one single lateralized brain region. Hence abnormalities of distributed functions do not, with a few notable exceptions, arise from small discrete lesions, but result from fairly extensive, and usually bilateral, damage. *Localized* functions are lateralized to one hemisphere, and often one part of a hemisphere. Localized functions can in turn be divided into those associated with the dominant, usually left, hemisphere, and those associated with the non-dominant hemisphere.

In this chapter I shall describe the three broad areas of cognition with a distributed neural basis: attention/concentration, memory, and higher-order frontal/executive function. This is followed by a brief discussion of delirium and the dementias. Chapter 2 covers the localized functions. The tests mentioned in Chapters 1 and 2 are described more fully in Chapter 4 and in the Appendix.

Table 1.1   Distributed cognitive functions

Cognitive function	Neural basis
1. Attention/concentration	Reticular activating system (brain stem and thalamic nuclei), and multimodal association areas (prefrontal, posterior parietal and temporal lobes)
2. Memory	Limbic system (especially hippocampus and diencephalon)
3. Higher-order intellectual functions, social behaviour, and personality	Frontal lobes

Attention/concentration

Although attention is extremely important, affecting performance in virtually all cognitive domains, it is difficult to state specific defining characteristics. 'Vigilance', 'concentration', and 'persistence' are used to describe the positive aspects of attention. A disturbance of attentional mechanisms causes impersistence, distractibility, increased vulnerability to interference, and difficulty in inhibiting immediate, but inappropriate, responses. Disorientation in time, and sometimes in place, is an inevitable consequence of disordered attention.

The clinical syndrome which exemplifies a disorder of attention is the acute confusional state (sometimes called acute organic psychiatric syndrome or delirium). Although other abnormalities are frequently found in acute confusional states, disordered attention is the principal and most consistent disturbance. Clouding of consciousness is often said to be the cardinal feature. However, attention is *not* synonymous with wakefulness, as many acutely confused patients do not demonstrate disturbed consciousness, and sleepy patients are not necessarily confused. This is discussed more fully in the section on delirium (see p. 25).

Applied anatomy

Maintenance of attention depends upon integrated activity of the neocortex (especially pre-frontal areas), thalamus, and brain stem. These structures are functionally linked by the reticular activating system (see Fig. 1.1). Components of this system in the brain stem are the reticular formation and adjacent nuclei (for example, the midline raphe, the nucleus of the locus coeruleus, and tegmental nuclei), which receive collaterals from a large number of ascending and descending pathways. This enables them to integrate a wide spectrum of neural information. These nuclei give rise to major ascending cholinergic, monoaminergic (for example, dopamine), and serotinergic pathways destined for the thalamus and cortical areas. The thalamus acts as a major relay station between the cortex and reticular formation: the intralaminar nuclei receive inputs from the brain stem nuclei and relay information widely to the cortex. A reciprocal feedback loop from the cortex modulates these ascending pathways via the thalamus. Thus the thalamus plays an essential role in regulating and integrating attentional mechanisms. The areas of the cortex most involved in these functions are the so-called 'higher-order multimodal association areas', which receive inputs from many primary sensory cortical and association areas and relay to the limbic system. The most important multimodal association areas are the pre-frontal, posterior parietal, and ventral temporal lobes. Of these, the frontal lobes are the most involved in attentional mechanisms. There is also evidence of asymmetrical function, since the cortical lesions causing severe confusional states are most commonly right-sided.

Thus disorders of attention may arise in conditions which disrupt the function of any of these three components: the reticular formation and the nuclei of the brain stem, the thalamic nuclei, and the pre-frontal cortex (especially on the right). The disruption may

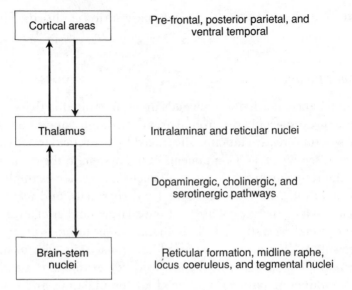

Fig. 1.1 Reticular activating system: major structures and pathways involved in normal attentional process.

result from a wide variety of structural causes, or, more commonly, from metabolic disorders and pharmacological agents affecting the ascending pathways (see 'causes of delirium', p. 31). A lesser degree of attentional impairment, without the other features of delirium, is seen in patients with focal lesions, involving particularly the frontal and right parietal lobes, and is also a fairly common accompaniment of diffuse brain injury.

Tests of attention/concentration (see Chapter 4 and Appendix for details)

1. Orientation in time and place (also dependent upon memory).

2. Digit span, especially digits backwards.

3. Recitation of the months of the year or the days of the week backwards.

4. Serial subtraction of 7s.

5. Timed letter or star cancellation tasks (also detect neglect phenomena, see p. 74).

Memory

Introduction

Neuropsychological research on humans and primates with focal brain lesions has shown that memory is not a single all-encompassing system. Unfortunately, a plethora of terms has arisen to describe the various subcomponents. One broad distinction divides memory into that available to conscious access and reflection (called **explicit** or **declarative memory**), and those types of learned responses, such as conditioned reflexes and motor skills, which are not available for conscious reflection (called **implicit** or **procedural memory**).

Explicit memory is further divided into two systems: one is responsible for the laying down and recall of personally experienced and highly temporally specific events or episodes—this is termed **episodic memory.** The other, responsible for out permanent store of representational knowledge of facts and concepts, as well as of words and their meanings, is termed **semantic memory.** Although in linguistics and philosophy 'semantics' refers purely to the study of word meaning, in cognitive psychology semantic memory has wider usage, and applies to our general store of world knowledge. Semantic memory is generally acquired early in life, but continues to expand, to variable degrees, throughout life. It is organized conceptually, without reference to the time and context in which it was acquired. Both episodic and semantic memory are components of our long-term memory systems (see Fig. 1.2).

To illustrate this further, recalling the details of a conversation earlier in the day or a holiday last year depends upon episodic memory. Knowing the meaning of the word 'perimeter', the capital of France, and the boiling-point of water, and being able to identify a small yellow bird as a canary, all depend on semantic memory. The content of both these stores is avaliable to conscious access. By contrast, the acquisition of motor skills, such as learning to drive a car or to play a musical instrument, does not use explicit memory, but relies upon a separate implicit memory system.

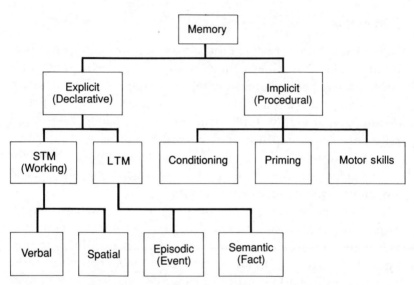

Fig. 1.2　Major subdivisions of memory (STM = Short-term memory; LTM = Long-term memory).

The term 'memory disorder' may, therefore, apply to various different types of problem. Most commonly, it is used to mean a disorder of episodic memory, that is to say difficulty in recalling personally experienced episodes from the past and/or learning new information. Disorders of episodic memory will be dealt with in more detail below. In brief, they occur either in the context of diffuse brain disease (as part of dementia), or as a result of selective damage to bilateral limbic structures, when the disorder is purer, sparing other aspects of cognition, and is termed the 'amnesic syndrome'.

Table 1.2 Divisions within long-term memory

	Type of material	Neural substrate
Explicit		
Episodic	• Personally experienced episodes and events. Time- and context-specific.	Limbic system
Semantic	• Vocabulary, facts, concepts, etc. Not time- and context-specific.	Temporal neocortex
Implicit		
Procedural	• Motor skills, e.g. driving, playing golf	Basal ganglia
	• Priming	Cerebral cortex
	• Classical conditioning	Unknown, cerebellar?

Semantic memory loss is also an integral part of most dementing illnesses. Isolated impairment of semantic memory is uncommon, but occasionally occurs following temporal neocortical damage. Implicit memory is preserved in the amnesic syndrome, but impaired in basal ganglia disorders such as Huntington's disease.

Short-term (working) memory

In neuropsychological terms, short-term memory is synonymous with the system of working memory responsible for the immediate recall of small amounts of verbal (as in, for example, digit span) or spatial material. It was traditionally held that for new information to enter long-term memory it must first pass through this short-term store. Likewise, it was believed that material recalled from long-term memory stores must first be processed by the immediate store. This simplistic model has been rejected by the discovery of brain-injured patients with defective short-term memory, yet completely normal ability to lay down and retrieve new longer-term memories. In addition, a number of apparently normal subjects (usually undergraduates who unwisely volunteered for psychology experiments!) have been found to have very limited short-term memory capacities. It is also worth noting at this point that patients with very severe deficits in forming new memories, as in Korsakoff's syndrome, have normal short-term memory.

There is now good evidence that there are, in fact, various subcomponents of **working memory** responsible for the immediate repetition of words, numbers, and melodies, etc. (called the phonological or articulatory loop), and for spatial information (called the visuo-spatial sketch pad) both of which are controlled by a central executive. Working memory appears to function independently of, but in parallel with, longer-term memory. The central executive component of working memory is associated with frontal lobe function and is particularly important for dual-task performance; the phonological loop depends upon peri-sylvian language areas in the dominant (left) hemisphere; and the visuo-spatial scratch pad is probably located in the non-dominant hemisphere. Hence damage to widely dispersed brain regions may impair distinct components of working memory. For example, a reduced digit is common in aphasic patients with left hemisphere lesions and in patients with frontal lobe dysfunction; but the mechanisms underlying this are different in the two instances. In the former, the phonological loop system is defective, while in the latter damage to the central executive is responsible.

Clinicians use 'short-term memory' loosely to refer to the recall of new material over an ill-defined short period, typically 5–30 minutes; but sometimes also to mean retention over days. There is no evidence, however, either from the study of normal controls or patients with memory disorders, to support a storage system with these characteristics. As we have seen above, the neuropsychological evidence points to there being one system which is responsible for very short-term (or immediate) recall of verbal or spatial material (termed working memory), and a number of long-term systems responsible for different types of material; episodic, semantic, procedural, etc. This brief discussion highlights the controversy over the term 'short-term memory'. To avoid the confusion surrounding this term, I have avoided as much as possible talking about short-term memory. When I do apply this term it is used in the neuropsychological sense, to mean 'immediate' or 'working' memory. In clinical practice, a much more useful distinction is between the acquisition of new information (**anterograde memory**) and the recall of previously learnt material (**retrograde memory**), since these two components may be impaired independently in different pathologies, as we shall see below.

Episodic memory

Applied anatomy

Extensive studies of patients with naturally occurring lesions and those who have undergone neurosurgery have established which structures are critical for the laying down and retrieval of episodic memories: the medial temporal structures (particularly the hippocampus, the parahippocampal gyrus, and the entorhinal cortex); the diencephalon (mamilliary bodies, and the anterior and dorsomedial nuclei of the thalamus and connecting tracts), which surrounds the third ventricle; and the basal forebrain nuclei (the septal nucleus, the diagonal band, the nucleus basalis). All of these are bilaterally represented. The principal areas are connected by a number of pathways, including the fornix and the cingulate gyrus. Together these structures constitute the limbic system, sometimes referred to as the circuit of Papez (see Fig. 1.3). The hippocampus has traditionally been viewed as the central component of this system. It receives afferents from, and sends efferents to, each of the sensory association areas (i.e., the visual, auditory, somatosensory, areas). The internal circuitry of the hippocampus has also been worked out in great detail; inputs arrive at the dentate gyrus via the

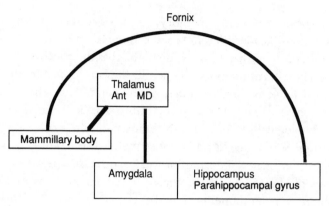

Fig. 1.3 Principal components of the limbic system concerned with episodic memory.

perforant pathway; the dentate gyrus then projects to the CA3 zone, which in turn projects to CA1; the latter relays to the subiculum, which sends efferents back to the association areas and to the mamilliary bodies via the fornix.

   Damage anywhere in the limbic system can produce memory deficits; but these are often subtle and material-specific. For instance, surgical removal or infarction of the left hippocampus produces a selective memory deficit for verbal material. In contrast, right-sided injury to the same structures causes specific non-verbal memory problems (for instance in learning faces and spatial information) that may not be apparent without detailed assessment. Bilateral damage to either the medial temporal regions or the diencephalon, however, produces a devastating and profound amnesic syndrome for both verbal and non-verbal material.

Disorders of episodic memory: transient amnesia; the amnesic syndrome

These occur in the context of diffuse injury, which may be either transient (acute confusional states or delirium) or chronic (dementia). In both of these syndromes the memory deficit is multifactorial, with contributions from decreased attention/concentration, impaired retrieval strategies, and defective memory *per se*. The term amnesic syndrome should be restricted to patients with a pure disorder of memory, sparing global intellectual functions. Such disorders may also be acute and transient, or chronic and generally permanent (see Table 1.3).

Transient amnesia   Transient global amnesia is an interesting and not uncommon disorder. It occurs typically in later life, with a peak around in the sixth and seventh decades. Cases below the age of forty are exceptional. The patient, who is generally in good health, suddenly becomes profoundly amnesic. Short-term (working) memory is preserved, but he or she is unable to retain any new information for more than a few seconds. The anterograde amnesia is accompanied by a variable retrograde amnesia for the past weeks, months, or even years. Patients appear disorientated and repetitively ask the same cycle of questions (for example, What's happened?'; 'Why am I here?' 'What day is it?'). But there is no impairment of attention or of consciousness, and no aphasia or visuo-spatial deficit. After a few hours the ability to lay down new memories returns, and the retrograde amnesia shrinks until patients are left with only a dense amnesic gap for the duration of the attack. Recurrence is unusual, and the general prognosis is excellent. The cause of this syndrome remains unknown. It is now clear that thrombo-embolic cerebrovascular disease does not play a role; but there is an association with migraine. A few cases go on to develop epilepsy of the temporal lobe type.

Closed head injury may cause a state very similar to transient global amnesia; but there is usually a very limited retrograde amnesia, and attentional processes are also often impaired.

Hysterical or psychogenic fugue states are now rare. They occur predominantly in young adults with a background of psychiatric problems, and there is usually a recognizable major precipitating life event (such as bereavement, separation, criminal charges, etc.). In contrast to transient global amnesia, there is a profound

Table 1.3　Causes of episodic memory impairment

	Pure amnesia	Mixed (other accompanying cognitive deficits)
Acute (transient)	Transient global amnesia Epilepsy (temporal lobe) Closed head injury Drugs—e.g. Benzoadiazepines 　　　　　　Alcohol Psychogenic (hysterical) fugues	Delirium (see p. 25)
Chronic (persistent)	Amnesic syndrome: 1. **Hippocampal damage** 　*Herpes simplex* virus 　　encephalitis 　Anoxia 　Surgical removal of temporal 　　lobes 　Bilateral posterior cerebral 　　artery occlusion 　Closed head injury 　Early Alzheimer's disease 2. **Diencephalic damage** 　Korsakoff's syndrome 　　(alcoholic and non- 　alcoholic) 　IIIrd ventricle tumours and 　　cysts 　Bilateral thalamic infarction 　Post subarachnoid 　　haemorrhage especially 　　from anterior 　　communicating artery 　　aneurysms	Dementia (see p. 33)

retrograde amnesia encompassing the subject's whole life, including a loss of personal identity, but often without significant anterograde memory impairment.

The amnesic syndrome: defining characteristics

1. *Preserved global intellectual abilities.* In alcoholic Korsakoff's syndrome subtle frontal lobe deficits are frequently present; but the sparing of general intellectual functions compared to memory should be very obvious clinically, and on neuropsychological testing. The gold standard is a significant discrepancy between the general Intelligence Quotient and the Memory Quotient.

2. *Anterograde amnesia*, i.e. severe impairment of the acquisition of new episodic memories.

3. *Retrograde amnesia*, i.e. impaired recall of past events. The degree depends to a large extent on the locus of damage, and hence the aetiology of the amnesic syndrome. Diencephalic amnesia, as exemplified by Korsakoff's syndrome, is characterized by temporally extensive retrograde amnesia covering many decades, with a pattern of relative preservation of more distant memories, called a temporal gradient. Hippocampal amnesia, by contrast, is accompanied by a much shorter retrograde amnesia (for months only).

4. *Preserved short-term/working memory* (for example, digit span).

5. *Preserved procedural (implicit) memory* (see p. 18).

The cognitive neuropsychology of the amnesic syndrome There is still considerable controversy about the basic cognitive deficit underlying the amnesic syndrome. Short-term (working) memory, as judged by digit span or registration of a name and address, is normal. According to contemporary information-processing accounts of memory the deficit in amnesia could be at any of the following stages:

(1) during the initial laying down (encoding) of new memories,

perhaps as a result of a defect in the normal time—and other contextual—labelling which is essential for subsequent retrieval;

(2) during the process which occur after initial encoding that are responsible for consolidation of long-term memory traces; or

(3) during the operation of memory retrieval.

Patients with diencephalic amnesia, as in Korsakoff's syndrome, have problems mainly with memory encoding, and hence lay down weak memory traces. Once information has entered into long-term stores there is no evidence of rapid decay or forgetting. However, patients with Korsakoff's syndrome also have an extensive and temporally graded retrograde amnesia. It has been argued that this remote memory deficit is due to the fact that alcoholics have been encoding weak memories for many years, because they spend their life in an alcohol-induced blur. A number of studies have refuted this suggestion, and it appears that retrieval *per se* is also defective in Korsakoff's syndrome. Moreover, exactly the same picture of severe anterograde and retrograde amnesia can be seen in patients with non-alcoholic (for example, stavation-induced) Korsakoff's syndrome, and in patients with bilateral thalamic infarcts. Hence there seems to be dual pathology, affecting the laying down of new memories, as well as the retrieval of both new and old memories, in diencephalic amnesia.

In hippocampal amnesia the situation is different; since remote memory is unaffected, a general retrieval deficit cannot be postulated. Opinions are divided as to whether the primary problem is one of encoding or of consolidation. There is only limited evidence for accelerated forgetting, suggesting that the main defect is in the laying down of new memories.

Memory impairment is also a major and early feature of Alzheimer's disease and other dementing disorders. In Alzheimer's the situation is even more complex than in the amnesic syndrome. Each of the processes involved in long-term memory—encoding, consolidation, and retrieval—may be impaired. One of the hallmarks of early Alzheimer's is a very rapid forgetting of any new material; but there is also an extensive retrograde amnesia, implying either problems with retrieval or a loss of stored information. Initially, short-term (working) memory may be normal; but with disease progression this too becomes defective. In addition, semantic memory breaks down, so that the patients' data-base of knowledge about the world progressively declines, leading to a range of deficits, including vocabulary, impaired word comprehension, and difficulty in naming objects.

Tests of anterograde episodic memory (see Appendix for details)

Verbal

- Recall of complex verbal information such as stories (for example, the logical memory subtest of the Wechsler Memory Scales and the Rivermead Behavioural Memory Test)

- Word-list learning (for example, the Rey Auditory Verbal Learning Test)

- Recognition memory for newly encountered words (for example, Warrington's Recognition Memory Test)

Non-verbal

- Recall of geometric figures (for example, the Rey–Osterrieth Figure Test, and the Visual Reproduction and Figural Memory subtests of the Wechsler Memory Scale)

- Recognition of newly encountered faces (for example, the Warrington Recognition Memory Test)

- Tests of spatial location recall (used in research projects)

Tests of Retrograde memory

Personal (autobiographical)

- The Autobiographical Memory Interview, which is a structured interview which probes for personal facts and episodes from three life-periods: school, early adult, and recent

- Cued word association (Galton–Crovitz technique), which tests for personally experienced episodes evoked by a standard test of words (for example, boat, train, baby, etc.), and is used in research projects on remote memory

Public events
- Famous Faces test, based on the identification and naming of photographs of personalities famous for a limited time in the past (for example, 1980s, 1970s, 1960s, etc.)

- Famous Events Tests, using either photographs or questionnaires about public events from various past eras.

Semantic memory

The storage, maintenance, and retrieval of factual information and vocabulary does not, in contrast to episodic memory, depend upon the limbic system. However, all new facts must presumably be acquired in the same way, via a common system. In other words, newly acquired facts are all initially episodic; but at some stage, perhaps with repeated rehearsal, they enter our fund of general knowledge. Their retrieval then becomes independent of the personal and time-tagged labels essential for recreating episodic memories. To illustrate this difference, consider attending a lecture on a new topic. Recall of the information is at first very dependent upon the context, and proceeds by reconstruction of the events at the time of acquisition. With repeated exposure (or retrievals) some of the information becomes part of our general store. Who can recall where and when they first learnt the meaning of the word haemorrhage, or the name of the capital of France?

The study of semantic memory is relatively recent; but current evidence points to the temporal neocortex, particularly in the left hemisphere, as the key region. A selective loss of semantic memory occurs as a result of extensive destruction of this region, often from *Herpes simplex* virus encephalitis, or occasionally vascular lesions. A generalized and progressive loss of semantic memory occurs in patients with Alzheimer's disease, who also have a severe impairment of episodic memory. Patients with circumscribed temporal lobe atrophy (Pick's disease) also have a dramatic loss of semantic memory. It seems that knowledge about certain categories of things is stored separately, and in a highly organized fashion. A growing number of patients have been reported with so-called 'category-specific' semantic memory loss, affecting for instance their knowledge about living rather than man-made things. Patients with even finer-grained deficits, involving for instance fruit and vegetables only, have also been reported.

Disorders of semantic memory

1. Selective impairment (i.e. sparing other cognitive abilities)
   - *Herpes simplex* virus encephalitis
   - Major head injury
   - Vascular lesions (for example, temporal lobe haemorrhage)
   - Focal temporal lobe atrophy (Pick's disease)

2. As part of more diffuse dementing disease
   - Alzheimer's disease

Tests of semantic memory (see Appendix for details)

1. Tests of general knowledge and vocabulary (for example, the Information, Similarities, and Vocabulary subtests of the Wechsler Adult Intelligence Scale)

2. Category fluency (i.e. generation of exemplars from specified semantic categories such as animals, fruit, etc.)

3. Object naming to confrontation, which also depends upon intact perceptual and word retrieval abilities (for example, the Boston Naming Test, the Graded Naming Test)

4. Picture-pointing in response to a spoken name

5. Tests of verbal knowledge (for example, 'What colour is a banana?'; 'Do canaries have wings?', etc.)

6. Non-verbal tests of semantic knowledge, such as those involving picture–picture matching (for example, the Pyramids and Palm Trees Test).

Implicit memory

Both episodic and semantic memory are available to conscious access. We can reflect on both personally experienced events and our fund of knowledge of the world. However, other forms of learning occur to which we do not have conscious access. These have been termed 'implicit' or 'procedural' memory. Consider the act of learning to play a musical instrument, or learning to drive a car. Although we progressively acquire the motor skills involved in these tasks, we cannot fully explain the procedures, and improvement can only be tested practically. Another form of implicit learning goes under the term **priming**—in this, exposure to test stimuli improves subsequent performance, even if the subject has no conscious recollection of the initial exposure. For instance, on word-stem completion tests, subjects are first shown a list of words (for example, TRACE, BREEZE, METER, etc.), then asked to recall the list, and finally shown the initial three letters of each word (TRA, BRE, MET, etc.) and asked to complete each stem with the first word that comes to mind. Amnesic patients do well on the last task, although they have no memory of having seen the words. In a non-verbal priming test, fragmented-picture identification, subjects are shown a series of progressively less fragmented pictures of the same object, and asked to say as soon as they recognize the object. Normal subjects identify the objects much sooner (ie. from more fragmented pictures) when re-shown the pictures. Amnesic patients demonstrate the same effect, although they deny having seen them before.

Implicit memory appears to depend neither upon the limbic

system nor upon the temporal neocortex. Even patients with profound amnesia (for example, Korsakoff's syndrome) have spared implicit memory. Current evidence points to the basal ganglia as the key region for motor learning, although priming appears to depend upon cortical areas, and the cerebellum may also be important for some classical conditioned responses.

Implicit memory is not testable at the bedside. Questioning may reveal preservation of practical skills in patients with severe impairment of explicit memory; but the main reason for its inclusion here is to make readers aware of this important and rapidly expanding area of neuropsychological investigation.

Higher-order cognitive function, personality, and behaviour

Introduction

The frontal lobes are undeniably crucial to the integrity of many aspects of 'higher-order' cognitive function, as well as to personality and behaviour. Damage to the pre-frontal areas produces long-lasting and often devastating deficits. Yet it is notoriously difficult to define these cognitive domains accurately. Furthermore, there are no really satisfactory bedside methods of assessment. Even the neuropsychological tests traditionally described as frontal lobe tasks are crude, and do not capture many of the behavioural aspects of frontal dysfunction. Here history taking from informants and clinical observation are especially important.

Cognitive functions attributed to the frontal lobes

- Adaptive behaviour

- Abstract conceptional ability

- Set-shifting/mental flexibility

- Problem-solving

- Planning

- Initiation

- Sequencing of behaviour

- Temporal-order judgements

- Personality, especially drive, motivation, and inhibition

- Social behaviour

Many of these aspects of cognition can be considered under the general headings of 'adaptive behaviour' and 'executive function': to be effective, behaviour must be appropriate, modifiable, motivated, and free from interference and disruptive impulsive responses. If responses are to be appropriately adapted, changes in the environment need to be monitored, and if possible anticipated. Patients with frontal lobe damage fail to anticipate changes, show poor planning ability, and do not learn from their errors. Planning is a particularly important practical function, since many complex behaviours—such as shopping, or holding down a job of work—require the planning and sequencing of behaviours, as well as the setting of goals. Frontal patients are especially poor at self-guided learning and goal-setting. They perform normally on externally driven tasks, but are very poor at self-motivated learning. There is a striking vulnerability to interference from irrelevant stimuli, resulting in distractibility and the intrusion of unwanted responses. They also show a tendency to perseverate. Perseveration can be observed on motor tasks (such as learning a sequence of hand movements, as in the Luria three-step test described on p. 121), when a compulsive repetition of movement is observed. Perseverative tendencies can also be seen on cognitive tests independent of motor activity, where subjects perseverate correct and incorrect responses. There is also an inability to shift from one task to another, and a peculiar mental stickiness described as 'stimulus-bound' behaviour. Many of the above cognitive functions are necessary for effective problem-solving; and it is, therefore, not surprising that frontal lobe damage results in severe deficits in solving problems, deducing concepts, and making analogies.

The inability to initiate cognitive strategies is tested by verbal fluency tasks. In the supermarket fluency test, patients are asked to list items which can be bought in a supermarket. In category fluency tests they are asked to list as many exemplars as possible from a given category (for example, animals, fruit, vegetables, etc.) in a limited time-period, usually one minute. Letter fluency tests require subjects to generate as many words as possible beginning with certain letters (for instance, F, A, and S). Frontal patients show severe impoverishment in the generation of exemplars, impaired search strategies, and a tendency to repeat the same item (see p. 219 for details of tests).

Although not involved in the laying down and storage of long-term memory traces, the frontal lobes are important for certain aspects of memory retrieval, particularly when temporal-order judgements are required. One of the components of working memory—the central executor—also depends critically upon the frontal lobes (see p. 8). Patients with frontal lobe dysfunction may, therefore, be impaired on simple tests of short-term (working) memory (for example, reverse digit span); but they show very marked deficits on dual-task performance tasks that place heavy demands upon working memory, such as simultaneous digit span and manual tracking.

One of the hallmarks of frontal lobe damage is loss of inhibitory control. This results in a tendency to react immediately, and usually inappropriately, to external stimuli. Irascibility and verbal aggression are common. The capacity to cope with personal relationships is frequently affected. A deterioration in social habits and hygiene may occur. A dulling of curiosity and vitality, and a loss of the capacity for empathy are common. Some patients may become inappropriately jocular and puerile. Many develop a peculiar anergia or passivity, which if profound results in a state of withdrawn akinetic mutism.

Frontal lobes: applied anatomy

The frontal lobes proper can be subdivided into five major areas (see Fig. 1.4):

(1) the motor area, which occupies the pre-central gyrus;

(2) the pre-motor area, which lies immediately anterior to the motor strip, and serves to co-ordinate and plan motor activity.

(3) the frontal eye fields, which mediate volitional and involuntary eye movements in the contralateral direction, and are also important for spatial attention;

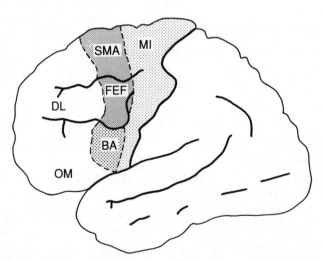

Fig. 1.4   The frontal lobes (M1 = primary motor cortex; SMA = supplementary motor area; FEF = frontal eye fields; BA = Broca's area; OM = orbito-medial; DL = dorsolateral pre-frontal area).

(4) Broca's area, which occupies the inferior pre-frontal region in the dominant, usually left, hemisphere; and

(5) the pre-frontal area proper.

In keeping with its role as the orchestrator of higher intellectual function, the pre-frontal cortex is richly connected with virtually all other cortical and sub-cortical structures. It receives inputs from all unimodal association areas (visual, auditory, etc.) and the other multimodal association areas (i.e. the posterior parietal and ventral temporal lobes), as well as from the limbic structures. Major afferent projections arise from the dorsomedial nucleus of the thalamus and basal ganglia. This accounts for the 'frontal lobe' deficits which typically occur in the subcortical dementia syndrome associated with basal ganglia disorders (for example, Huntington's disease, progressive supranuclear palsy, and Parkinson's disease), and in lesions of the thalamus.

From a clinical viewpoint, a division into lateral and orbitomedial (basomedial) regions has frequently been made. Changes in personality, behaviour, and motivation are associated with orbitomedial damage, while the dorsolateral region is more important for adaptive or executive behaviour, i.e. planning, sequencing, problem-solving, set-shifting, etc.

Disorders of frontal-lobe function

Degenerative
• Dementia of frontal type secondary to focal lobar atrophy (Pick's disease)

Vascular
• Bilateral anterior cerebral artery infarction
• Following subarachnoid haemorrhage (anterior communicating artery aneurysms)

Structural
• Major closed head injury

- Tumours (butterfly glioma and subfrontal meningioma)
- Surgical resection
- Frontal leucotomy

Deafferentation from basal ganglia disorders, for example:
- Huntington's disease
- Advanced Parkinson's disease
- Progressive supranuclear palsy (Steel–Richardson–Olzewski syndrome)
- Wilson's disease

Tests of frontal-lobe function (see Chapter 4 and Appendix for details)

- Verbal fluency (category and letter-based tests)

- Analogies and sequencing (for example, the Similarities and Picture Arrangement subtests from the WAIS, and Raven's Matrices)

- Proverb interpretation

- Cognitive Estimates Test

- Trail Making Test

- Card-sorting (for example, the Wisconsin Card Sorting Test)

- Motor sequencing (for example, alternating hand movements and the Luria three-step test)

- Problem-solving (for example, the Tower of London [or Hanoi] test, which requires subjects to move coloured discs on three posts to obtain target designs in a set number of moves)

Having considered the three major areas of cognition with a distributed neural basis—attention, memory, and executive function—this is an appropriate place to include a brief description of delirium and dementia, which almost invariably affect one or more of these cognitive domains. Although this is not meant to be a textbook of neurology or psychiatry, I have included brief descriptions of these syndromes, as patients with one, or both, of these constitute the commonest presentation in behavioural neurology and in old age psychiatry.

Delirium

Delirium may be defined as a transient organic mental syndrome of acute onset, characterized by marked attentional abnormalities, an impairment in global cognitive functions, perceptual disturbances, increased and/or decreased psychomotor activity, a disordered sleep–wake cycle, and a tendency to marked fluctuations.

Several components of this definition deserve further comment. Although delirium is a syndrome with certain core characteristics, the clinical manifestations may vary widely. The features vary between patients, and often in a single patient over the course of 24 hours. The onset is always acute or subacute, occurring over hours or days, and often at night. The total duration rarely exceeds weeks. The prognosis clearly depends upon the aetiology; but if the underlying cause is cured then a complete recovery can be expected. The aspects of cognition principally involved are those with a distributed cerebral basis—attention, memory, and higher-order executive functions (for example, planning, problem-solving, abstraction, sequencing, etc.). Deficits of the more localized cognitive functions, such as language and praxis, may also be seen; but the distributed-function deficits always dominate. Clouding of consciousness is no longer included in contemporary definitions of delirium, for the reasons discussed below.

Features of delirium (acute confusional state)

1. Reduced ability to maintain attention to external stimuli, and to shift attention to new stimuli appropriately

2. Disorganized thinking, as indicated by rambling, irrelevant, or incoherent speech

3. Memory impairment: poor registration and retention of new material

4. Perceptual distortions, leading to misidentification, illusions, and hallucinations

5. Increased or decreased psychomotor activity

6. A disturbed sleep–wake cycle

7. Disorientation in time, and often in place

8. Changes in mood, such as anxiety, depression, or lability

9. A tendency to fluctuations and nocturnal exacerbation

Attention and memory

A disturbance in attention is the most striking and consistent abnormality: patients are unable to generate and sustain attention to external stimuli, and have problems with shifting attention appropriately. They appear distractible, and easily lose the thread of conversations. Accordingly, there is severe impairment on tests requiring sustained concentration and the manipulation of material, such as serial subtraction of 7s, recitation of the months of the year or days of the week in reverse order, and digit span. Another good test to sustained attention is ability to generate words beginning with certain letters (for example, F, A, and S) or from specific semantic categories (for example, animals, fruit, etc.). Patients with impaired attention produce few exemplars, tend to perseverate, and revert to a previous category.

Disorientation in time is almost always present at some time during the illness. Disturbed appreciation of the passage of time is universal. Disorientation for place, and still later for person, may follow with worsening of perceptual and cognitive organization.

The disturbance in memory is largely secondary to diminished attention. Incoming sensory material is poorly attended to and registered. Immediate repetition of a name and address is characteristically defective, and patients need multiple presentations before simple material is repeated correctly. Confabulatory responses may be seen. Retrograde memory is reasonably intact if the patient's attention can be focused and sustained. On recovery from delirium there is typically a dense amnesic gap for the period of the illness, although where fluctuation has been marked islands of memory may remain.

Thinking

The organization and content of thought processes are invariably affected in delirium. Even in mild cases there is difficulty in formulating complex ideas and sustaining a logical train of thought. Attempts at history taking reveal the muddled, illogical, and disjointed nature of the patient's thinking. The capacity to select thoughts and maintain their organization and sequence for the purpose of problem-solving and planning is drastically reduced. Concept-formation is impaired, with a tendency to concrete thinking. These deficits are apparent on bedside testing of proverb interpretation, similarity judgement, generation of word definitions, and category fluency.

The content of thought may be dominated by the patient's concerns, wishes, and fantasies. There is often a dream-like quality to the patient's thinking. Delusions (i.e. false beliefs incongruent with the patient's cultural and educational background) are often present. These are usually fleeting, poorly elaborated, and inconsistent. A paranoid persecutory content is most common. For instance, patients may believe that they are about to be killed by the nurse or doctors, or that close family members have been murdered. Delusions, illusions, and hallucinations frequently occur together.

Disorders of perception

Perception in this context refers to the ability to extract information from the environment and one's own body and to integrate it in a meaningful way. Attentional processes play a crucial role in the perception of sensory information, and the ubiquitous attentional disorder seen in delirium probably underlies many of the perceptual disturbances seen. Vision and hearing are most commonly affected. Disturbance of vision may lead to micropsia, macropsia, or distortions of shape and position, fragmentation, apparent movement, or autoscopy (the perception of seeing oneself from outside the body). Sounds may be accentuated or distorted. Body image may be affected, causing a perceived alteration of size, shape, or position. Bizarre reduplicative phenomena may be reported—for example, when the patient perceives the presence of two heads on one body. Feelings of depersonalization and unreality are very common.

Illusions—the misperception of external stimuli—are frequent, and most often involve the visual modality. Patients may mistake spots on the wall for insects, or patterns on the bed-cover for snakes. Illusions may be interwoven with delusions, so that ward sounds are incorporated into persecutory plots. Family members and staff may be misidentified.

Hallucinations are also common. Visual hallucinations are most characteristic, and range in complexity from simple shapes and patterns to fully formed objects, animals, mythological or ghostlike apparitions, and panoramic scenes. They are often brightly coloured, with elements that change in position, size, and number. The hallucinated material may be grossly distorted, as for example in Lilliputian hallucinations, where minute people or objects appear. Combined auditory and visual hallucinations are also frequent. Tactile hallucinations take the form of crawling, creeping, or burning sensations. Delusions of infestation or sexual interference may accompany such sensations. Olfactory hallucinations are also described. In general, hallucinations occur in patients with the hyperalert variant of delirium. Withdrawal from alcohol and sedative-hypnotics seems particularly prone to produce frank hallucinosis.

The sleep–wake cycle

A disruption of the normal saccadian sleep–wake cycle is a consistent feature of delirium, and is considered by some authors to be central to the pathogenesis of the syndrome. Insomnia, with a worsening of confusion at night, is common. Other features include daytime sleepiness, dreamlike states with vivid imagery, and a breakdown in the ability to distinguish between dreams and reality.

EEG tracings taken during the day show fluctuations, and transition from wakefulness, light, REM, and deep sleep. Night-time recordings show a loss of the normal orderly progression of the stages of sleep. Maintenance of the normal sleep–wake cycle depends upon the complex interaction of neurotransmitter systems that constitute the reticular activating system (see p. 3).

Psychomotor behaviour, emotion, and mood

A disturbance of general psychomotor activity is virtually always present in delirium. Two contrasting patterns may be distinguished; but not infrequently patients alternate between the two.

In the *hyperalert* variant, the patient is restless, excitable, and vigilant. He or she responds promptly, and often excessively, to any stimulus. Speech is voluble and pressured. Shouting, laughing, and crying are common. There is increased physical activity, and repetitive purposeless behaviour, such as groping or picking. Often the patient tries to get out of bed, and attempts at restraint may produce violent outbursts. Autonomic signs of hyperarousal, such as tachycardia, sweating, and pupillary dilatation can be observed. Vivid hallucinations tend to be seen most often in patients with this variant.

Patients with the *hypoalert* variant are, by contrast, quiet and motionless; they drift off to sleep if unstimulated, and display reduced psychomotor activity. Speech is typically sparse and slow; answers to questions are stereotypes, and often incoherent. Despite outward appearances the patient may be experiencing delusions and hallucinations, although they are less frequent than in the hyperalert variant.

Emotional disturbances are very frequent, and may vary from euphoria to depression. A state of perplexity, with apathy and indifference, is perhaps most often seen. Lability is common, and the patient may suddenly become fearful, angry, and aggressive.

Clouding of consciousness

This term was traditionally included in descriptions of delirium, but has been dropped from current definitions. There is no generally accepted definition of consciousness; and 'clouding' is an even vaguer term. Consciousness may be considered in a narrow sense to mean a level of wakefulness and response to gross external stimuli. Although patients with delirium may be drowsy and show reduced response when stimulated, often they are fully awake, and may even be hyperalert. In a broader sense, consciousness has been used to describe the capacity to engage in complex and appropriate thought, to fix, sustain, and shift attention, and to judge the passage of time. Impairment or clouding of consciousness, used in this sense, is thus no more than a metaphor referring to the set of cognitive and attentional deficits that constitute the core of the syndrome of delirium.

Causes of delirium (acute confusional states)

1. Metabolic encephalopathies
   - Acid–base or electrolyte imbalance
   - Hypoglycaemia
   - Hypoxia, hypercapnia
   - Hepatic or renal failure
   - Wernick's encephalopathy and other B-vitamin deficiencies
   - Endocrine disorders, for example Cushing's disease, Addison's disease
   - Porphyria

2. Intoxication by drugs and poisons
   - A wide range of drugs, including anticholinergics, hypnotic-sedatives, anti-parkinsonian agents, anticonvulsants, digoxin, etc.
   - Alcohol, illicit drugs, and inhalants
   - Industrial poisons

3. Withdrawal syndromes, especially alcohol and hypnotic-sedatives.

4. Infections, both intracranial (meningitis, encephalitis) and systemic

5. Multifocal and diffuse brain disease
   - Anoxia, fat embolism
   - Vasculitis
   - Cerebrovascular disease
   - Raised intracranial pressure, hydrocephalus

6. Head trauma

7. Epilepsy, including post-ictal states and non-convulsive status

8. Focal brain lesions, particularly to the brain stem or right hemisphere

Table 1.4 Differential diagnosis of delirium and dementia

Feature	Delirium	Dementia
Onset	Acute, often at night	Insidious
Course	Fluctuating, with lucid intervals during the day; worse at night	Stable over the course of the day
Duration	Hours to weeks	Months or years
Awareness	Reduced	Clear
Alertness	Abnormally low or high	Usually normal
Attention	Impaired, causing distractibility; fluctuation over the course of the day	Relatively unaffected
Orientation	Usually impaired for time; tendency to mistake unfamliar places and persons	Impaired in later stages
Short-term (working) memory	Always impaired	Normal in early stages
Episodic memory	Impaired	Impaired
Thinking	Disorganized, delusional	Impoverished
Perception	Illusions and hallucinations, usually visual and common	Absent in earlier stages, common later
Speech	Incoherent, hesitant, slow or rapid	Difficulty in finding words
Sleep–wake cycle	Always disrupted	Usually normal

Dementia

The term 'dementia' has traditionally been applied to a syndrome of acquired global impairment of intellectual function which is usually progressive, and occurs in a setting of clear consciousness. As we have seen above, clouding of consciousness was considered a hallmark of delirium; but because of definitional problems it has been removed from more recent criteria. The defining characteristics of delirium are now the disturbed attentional abilities and disordered thinking, which are not seen in dementia. The adjective 'acquired' is included to distinguish dementia from congenital or early-life intellectual impairment (mental handicap). The main conceptual development in recent years, however, has been to refine the meaning of 'global impairment of intellectual function', so that dementing disorders can now be diagnosed earlier, and with greater accuracy. Although a global or diffuse loss of higher cerebral function is the eventual fate of patients with dementia, the majority (if not all) cases begin with more circumscribed cognitive impairment. Modern definitions—such as that used in the Diagnostic and Statistic Manual of Mental Disorders (DSM III-R)—are more specific, and require:

1. Impairment of two or more of the following areas to cognition, sufficient to interfere with work, social function, or relationship:
   - Memory, which is virtually always affected
   - Language
   - Abstract thinking and judgement
   - Praxis
   - Visuo-spatial or perceptual skills
   - Personality
   - Social conduct

2. The absence of features of delirium.

3. The exclusion of non-organic psychiatric disorders, for example major depression or schizophrenia.

Causes of dementia

Common causes

- Alzheimer's disease
- Multi-infarct disease
- Focal lobar atrophy (Pick's disease)
- Parkinson's disease and diffuse cortical Lewy body disease
- Huntington's disease

Treatable causes

- Depressive pseudodementia
- Benign tumours, especially subfrontal meningiomas
- Normal pressure hydrocephalus
- Subdural haematoma
- Deficiency states—B_1, B_{12}, B_6
- Endocrine disease—hypothyroidism, Cushing's disease, Addison's disease
- Infections—AIDS dementia complex, syphilis
- Alcoholic dementia
- Wilson's disease

Other rare or untreatable causes

- Degenerative disorders, progressive supranuclear palsy (Steel–Richardson–Olzewski syndrome), striatonigral degeneration, etc.
- Non-metastatic syndrome of carcinoma (limbic encephalitis)
- Creutzfeldt–Jakob disease
- Progressive multifocal leucoencephalopathy (PML)
- Subacute sclerosing panencephalitis (SSPE)

Cortical versus subcortical dementia

A recently proposed division of primary degenerative diseases, which has proved theoretically and practically useful, is between those which affect primarily the cerebral cortex and those in which the major pathological impact is on subcortical structures. The reason for the cognitive impairment in the former is obvious. In the subcortical dementias, the major impact is thought to result from a loss of the normal regulatory effect of subcortical structures on the cortex, particularly the pre-frontal area. The term subcortical dementia was initially applied to the cognitive syndrome seen in progressive supranuclear palsy and Huntington's disease, but has been subsequently applied to a range of basal ganglia and white matter diseases.

Table 1.5 Cortical and subcortical dementias

Cortical dementias	Subcortical dementias
Alzheimer's disease	Progressive supranuclear palsy (Steele–Richardson–Olzewski syndrome)
Creutzfeldt–Jakob disease	Huntington's disease
	Parkinson's disease
	Wilson's disease
	Normal pressure hydrocepalus
	White matter diseases (leucodystrophies and multiple sclerosis)
	AIDS encephalopathy

Alzheimer's disease is the prototypical example of a cortical dementia in which disturbances of memory, language, praxis, and visuo-spatial abilities predominate. Attention and frontal executive functions are relatively well preserved. The slowing of cognitive processes (bradyphrenia), change in personality, and mood disturbances which characterize subcortical dementias are not seen, at least in the early stages of the disease. Marked impairment in episodic memory is practically always the earliest feature in Alzheimer's disease. The amnesia reflects a failure of encoding and a very rapid forgetting of any new material. Recall and recognition are both severely affected. Remote memory is also affected, with a temporal gradient, in that early-life memories are relatively spared. Within the domain of language, aphasia occurs fairly early in the course; the aphasia reflects a breakdown in the semantic components of language, with relative sparing of phonology and syntax; word-finding difficulty in spontaneous conversation, impaired naming on formal tests, and impaired generation of exemplars on category fluency testing (for example, on animals, or fruit) are consistent early findings; the picture in more advanced Alzheimer's disease has been likened to transcortical sensory aphasia (see p. 59). Visuo-spatial deficits are also obvious from fairly early in the course of the disease.

In subcortical dementia, as exemplified by Huntington's disease or progressive supranuclear palsy, impairment in attentional control and frontal 'executive' function predominate. Patients appear characteristically 'slowed up' (bradyphrenic), with a marked deficit in the retrieval of information. Spontaneous speech is reduced, and answers to questions are slow and laconic. Changes in mood, personality, and social conduct are very common. Patients are often inert, indifferent, and uninterested. Memory is impaired, mainly as a result of reduced attention, and hence poor encoding of new material; but the severe amnesia which typifies Alzheimer's disease is not seen in the early stages. Recognition is typically much better than spontaneous recall. It is easy to overestimate the degree of cognitive impairment in patients with subcortical dementia, and performance usually improves with persistence. Features of focal cortical dysfunction, such as aphasia, apraxia, and agnosia, are characteristically absent, at least in the earlier stages. But visuo-spatial and perceptual abnormalities can be demonstrated fairly consistently.

It should be pointed out that not all dementias can be fitted neatly into this dichotomy. In multi-infarct dementia, for example, subcortical features predominate, owing to multiple lacunar lesions in the basal ganglia and deep white matter; but there is often evidence of focal cortical damage.

Another recently identified disease in which a mixture of cortical and subcortical features occur is diffuse cortical Lewy body disease. The pathological hallmark of Parkinson's disease is the presence of Lewy bodies in the substantia nigra. In diffuse cortical Lewy body disease, as the term implies, the inclusion bodies are found throughout the cortex. Patients display a mixed picture with characteristic subcortical deficits, and features of cortical dysfunction, the latter particularly implicating posterior parieto-occipital regions. Visual hallucinations and misidentification phenomena are common. There is often a fluctuating course, with nocturnal confusion. Even small doses of anti-parkinsonian and neuroleptic drugs are liable to precipitate confusion, with prominent hallucinations.

Alzheimer's disease

Although initially considered to be a rare cause of pre-senile dementia, it is now clearly established that Alzheimer's disease is the commonest cause of dementia at all ages, and that its prevalence rises dramatically with advancing years. The distinction between pre-senile and senile dementia is, in general, no longer valid. The defining characteristic of Alzheimer's disease remains the neuro-pathology, which consists of intraneuronal tangles of paired helical filaments and extraneuronal plaques containing an amyloid core. Since there is no definitive way of establishing the diagnosis in life, it has become common practice to apply the term dementia of Alzheimer type (DAT). However, with the use of strict research criteria (such as the NINCDS–ADRDA) an accurate diagnosis can be made in at least 80 per cent of cases. Alzheimer's disease does not

Table 1.6 Summary of features of cortical and subcortical dementias

Function	Cortical dementia (e.g. Alzheimer's disease)	Subcortical dementia (e.g. Huntington's disease)
Alertness	Normal	Marked 'slowing up' (bradyphrenia)
Attention	Intact in early stages	Impaired
Episodic memory	Severe amnesia	Forgetfulness due to poor encoding; recognition better than recall
Frontal 'executive' function	Normal until late	Typically impaired from onset
Personality	Preserved	Apathetic, inert
Language	Aphasic features	Normal, except for reduced output and dysarthria
Praxis	Impaired	Normal
Visuo-spatial and perceptual abilities	Impaired	Impaired

begin with a 'global' loss of intellectual function, but generally progresses in a predictable fashion through the following stages.

Stage 1: Even from the onset there is severe memory impairment, with features that are indistinguishable from those resulting from other causes of the amnesic syndrome (see p. 12). Anterograde amnesia results from poor encoding and rapid forgetting of new material. The retrograde memory loss has a temporally graded pattern, with sparing of more distant memories. Short-term (working) memory as judged by digit span is generally normal. Since attentional mechanisms remain intact, patients are often well orientated at this stage. Language is typically normal on informal assessment, but mild anomia on formal naming tests and poor generation of exemplars on category fluency (for example in naming animals, fruit, etc.) may be found. Visuo-spatial functioning is good on simple bedside assessment, although deficits are often apparent on formal testing. Social rapport and personality are well preserved.

Stage 2: Worsening memory abilities and impaired attention result in marked temporal disorientation. Impairment in short-term (working) memory is found. Distractibility and problems with frontal executive function occur. Breakdown of semantic memory results in diminished vocabulary, word-finding difficulty, and semantic paraphasic errors in spontaneous conversation, very poor naming ability, reduced generation of exemplars on category fluency testing, and a loss of general knowledge. Marked visuo-spatial and perceptual deficits are readily apparent. Hallucinations and delusions may arise at this stage. Social rapport is still generally intact, and because of this patients appear superficially to be reasonably intact; but beneath the social veneer they are empty shells.

Stage 3: Marked global loss in all areas of intellectual function—amnesia, aphasia, agnosia, etc. There is also progressive disintegration of personality. Disorders of social conduct and aggressive behaviour are common. Eventually incontinence and increasing dependence lead to death.

Focal lobar atrophy (Pick's disease)

Arnold Pick, a contemporary of Alois Alzheimer, recognized at the turn of the century the existence of a syndrome of progressive atrophy confined, at least initially, to either the frontal or temporal lobes. The characteristic pathological changes, distinct from that seen in Alzheimer's disease—ballooned cortical neurones (Pick cells) with argyrophilic inclusions (Pick bodies)—were subsequently identified, although these histological changes are not present in all cases. Pick's disease was considered to be a rare cause of dementia, largely indistinguishable from Alzheimer's disease; but the resurgence of interest in cognitive disorders and improved diagnostic tests have led to an increased recognition of cases of focal lobar atrophy. It has been claimed that 10–20 per cent of younger patients (i.e. of those below seventy) with cognitive impairment may have Pick's disease; but these estimates tend to be based on selected hospital-based series. The genetic component has been over-emphasized; the majority of cases are sporadic, although there are well-documented families with a dominant pattern of inheritance.

The clinical features depend upon the lobe involved.

Frontal lobe atrophy

This may present as either a loss of executive and social function, causing a so-called *dementia of frontal type*, or a *progressive non-fluent aphasia*. Often features of the two are combined. In dementia of frontal type, all the phenomena associated with frontal dysfunction can be observed (see p. 19). Often changes in personality and social conduct predominate. In the progressive aphasia subtype, there is a gradual decline in language abilities, affecting predominantly output, with a disintegration of grammar and phonology, which may progress to a state of complete mutism. The language disorder resembles a Broca's type aphasia, although syntax is often reasonably well preserved (see p. 55). In the early stages, comprehension is also relatively preserved, but often declines as the aphasia worsens.

Temporal lobe atrophy

The most common presentation of this subgroup is with word-finding difficulty and a reduced vocabulary, causing progressive aphasia, which differs from the non-fluent aphasic syndrome described above. Most of the features elicited on examination are explicable in terms of a breakdown in semantic memory (see p. 16) leading to severe anomia, impaired performance on category fluency tests, defective word–picture matching, and a loss of general knowledge. Speech remains fluent, with paraphasic errors and circumlocutions. The term **semantic dementia** has been applied to this syndrome. Episodic memory, and visuo-spatial and frontal executive abilities are usually preserved in the early stages, which contrasts sharply with the typical presenting features of Alzheimer's disease. As the disease progresses, patients may develop the *Kluver–Bucy syndrome*, as a result of bilateral damage to the amygdala. The features of this syndrome are a disturbance in eating behaviour, with a tendency to consume inedible things and a loss of satiety, increased libido, passivity, and usually severe associative visual agnosia.

Multi-infarct dementia

This term has replaced the older one, 'atherosclerotic dementia'. It occurs as a result of multiple infarcts, of varying size, caused by thrombo-embolism from extracranial arteries or small-vessel disease in the brain. There is usually, but not invariably, a history of stroke or transient ischaemic attacks. Vascular risk factors, especially hypertension, are readily apparent, and many patients have other evidence of atheromatous vascular disease (angina, claudication, cervical bruits, etc.). Cognitively, impaired attention and frontal features predominate, owing to a concentration of small vascular lesions (lacunes) in the basal ganglia and thalamic regions; but features of cortical dysfunction are also frequently present. Fluctuations in performance and night-time confusion are very common. Emotional lability, with other features of pseudobulbar palsy, is characteristic. There may be a step-wise progression, with periods of deterioration followed by more stable periods.

Huntington's disease

This genetic disorder is inherited in an autosomal dominant pattern, and has a negligible new mutation rate. A positive family history is, therefore, a requirement for diagnosis. In apparently *de novo* cases, it is necessary to question several family members to search for clues, such as a family history of psychiatric illness, suicide, dementia, or movement disorders.

Huntington's disease may present with psychiatric, neuropsychological, or neurological symptoms. The peak age of presentation is in the forties, but the age of presentation can be as late as seventy. Depression is common; but a schizophrenic-like state with paranoid delusions may also occur. An insidious change in personality, with the development of sociopathic behaviour, is very characteristic. Suicide is a frequent cause of death. The neuropsychological picture is one of subcortical dementia, with marked impairment on tests of attention and frontal function. Patients are forgetful because of impaired attention, but do not show marked amnesia. Language is preserved until late in the course. Visuo-perceptual deficits also occur fairly consistently.

The earliest sign of the movement disorder is a restless fidgetiness of the limbs, which the patient may learn to disguise. Eventually the chorea affects the face and extremities. The gait becomes unsteady and reeling. On walking, characteristic finger-flicking movements may be observed.

Pseudodementia

This term has been used to describe two rather distinct clinical syndromes: hysterical pseudodementia and depressive pseudodementia. The latter is more common, and is undoubtedly the most important treatable cause of memory failure.

Patients with *hysterical pseudodementia* usually present with a fairly abrupt onset of memory and intellectual loss. They typically appear unconcerned. Unlike organic amnesic disorders, the memory impairment is often worse for very salient personal and early-life events. Loss of personal identity may be seen. Memory is strikingly worse when being tested than during informal conversation about recent events. There is usually an identifiable precipitant (such as bereavement, marital problems, or offending) and a past psychiatric history. Patients may show features of the so-called *Ganser's syndrome*, the core symptom of which is the giving of 'approximate answers'. For example, when asked 'How many legs does a cow have?', they answer 'three', or in response to 'What is two plus two?' they reply 'five'. Another classic question is 'What colour is an orange?'! As in other hysterical conversion states, there may be an underlying organic disorder, which has been grossly exaggerated at either a conscious or a subconscious level.

Depressive pseudodementia is, on the whole, a condition of the elderly. Patients present complaining of poor memory or concentration, and deny overt depression. Clues to the diagnosis are biological features of depression, especially disturbed sleeping, low energy, psychomotor retardation, pessimistic and ruminative thoughts, and a lack of interest in activities and hobbies. The onset of the memory failure is usually relatively acute or subacute. A past or family history of affective illness may be an important marker. On bedside cognitive testing, attention is impaired, and performance on memory and executive tasks is patchy and often inconsistent. Typically, digit span and registration of a name and address are poor, but with repeated trials improve; and there is not the rapid forgetting of information seen in Alzheimer's disease. Responses on memory and other cognitive tests are frequently 'don't knows'. Language output is often slow and sparse, but paraphasic errors are not seen. Naming may elicit 'don't know' responses rather than other types of error. In some cases, however, it may be impossible to distinguish true dementia from pseudodementia on simple cognitive tests. If *any* of the above symptoms or signs are present a psychiatric opinion and a formal neuropsychological evaluation must be sought.

2. *Localized cognitive functions*

The functions ascribed to the dominant, usually left, cerebral hemisphere show much more clear-cut laterality than those associated with the so-called 'minor hemisphere'. This applies particularly to spoken language. Since language is such an important component of human cognition, and aphasia frequently complicates both focal and diffuse degenerative brain disease, I have dedicated a relatively large section to discussing aspects of normal and abnormal language function. There follows a brief description of disorders of calculation (acalculia) and of higher-order motor control (apraxia).

The second half of the chapter deals with disturbed right hemisphere functions: neglect phenomena, dressing and constructional apraxia, and complex visuo-perceptual deficits (agnosias).

Localized cognitive functions

A. *Dominant hemisphere*
  1. Language—most aspects of spoken language (phonology, semantics, syntax), plus reading and writing

  2. Calculation

  3. Praxis (higher motor control)

B. *Non-dominant hemisphere*
  1. Spatially-directed attention

  2. Complex visuo-perceptual skills

  3. Constructional abilities

  4. Prosodic components of language (tone, melody, intonation)

  5. Attention/concentration and vigilance (see Chapter 1)

Language

The general outline of this section is as follows.

1. Definitions and causes of aphasia and mutism.

2. Cerebral dominance, aspects of applied anatomy, and the role of the minor hemisphere.

3. Neurolinguistics made simple: a brief coverage of phonology, semantics, and syntax, plus the dual-route hypothesis of reading and writing.

4. The principles of classifying aphasic syndromes.

5. A description of the commoner syndromes: Broca's, Wernicke's, transcortical motor and sensory, and anomic aphasia.

6. Disorders of reading—the dyslexias.

7. Disorders of writing—the dysgraphias.

Aphasia is defined as a loss or impairment of language function caused by brain damage. Language should be separated from speech, since the two may be damaged independently. Speech is the term applied to co-ordinated muscle activity of oral communication and to the neural control of this activity; language is the complex symbolic signal system used by individuals to comunicate with one another. Clearly language is not only a spoken system, as communication occurs by reading and writing, and these functions may break down independently, to produce alexia or agraphia, respectively. Language disorders may also be observed in the congenitally mute who use sign language.

(*Note:* the terms aphasia and dysphasia are used interchangeably, even although technically aphasia should mean loss of language function and dysphasia should refer to a disturbance of language. The same applies to the terms alexia and dyslexia, and to the terms agraphia and dysgraphia.)

Disturbances of articulatory processes arise from a variety of pathologies involving peripheral speech mechanisms, as in bulbar palsy, and in cerebellar and basal ganglia deficits. Dysarthria frequently accompanies acute anterior left hemisphere lesions, but may also occur with acute right-sided lesions. Thus dysarthria and aphasia may coexist, but one is often seen without the other. Mutism is a complete failure of speech output which, if acquired, usually signifies either a severe language disorder or an articulation disorder, although occasionally mutism may be seen in psychiatrically ill patients.

Causes of aphasia

Focal lesions

- Strokes, usually middle cerebral artery territory infarcts or haemorrhages

- Tumours, either intrinsic (for example, gliomas, metastases) or extrinsic (for example meningiomas)

- Trauma

- Abscess

- Other rather space occupying lesions, tuberculomas, etc.

Dementias (but these rarely cause classical syndromes)

- Alzheimer's disease

- Focal lobar atrophy (Pick's disease) etc. (see p. 39)

Causes of mutism

1. *Strokes*
   - Acute global aphasia (middle cerebral artery strokes) accompanied by severely impaired comprehension, reading, and writing

   - Acute Broca's aphasia
     comprehension relatively normal
     writing may be unaffected

2. *Disorders of articulation: language comprehension and writing normal*
   - Bulbar palsy (lower motor neurone)
   - Pseudobulbar palsy (upper motor neurone)
3. *Psychiatric disorders*
   - Schizophrenia
   - Severe depression
   - Hysterical aphonia
   - Elective mutism

Dominance

The left hemisphere is strongly dominant for language functions in most humans. Therefore aphasia very rarely complicates right hemisphere damage in individuals who write with their right hand; when this does occur it is referred to as 'crossed aphasia'. The functional dominance has anatomical parallels; the superior part of the temporal lobe, the planum temporale, is consistently larger on the left side. The situation in left-handers is more complicated; a commonly stated figure for left hemisphere dominance in these individuals is around 50–60 per cent. In fact, most people who do *not* show a strong preference for writing with their right hand are, to some degree, ambidextrous. Commensurate with this, their language functions are more equally divided between the two hemispheres.

Applied anatomy

Within the left hemisphere, the area of supreme importance for language comprehension and production is the posterior superior temporal lobe (Wernicke's area). Deficits in this area consistently produce gross problems with the decoding of spoken and written language, and in the assembly of correct language output. The other major language area is in the inferior frontal lobe (Broca's and surrounding areas). Lesions here produce faltering, non-fluent, and distorted language output, with simplified or disturbed grammatical structure, although the comprehension of spoken and written language is largely intact. These two major areas are connected by means of the arcuate fasciculus; lesions here classically cause conduction aphasia, although this syndrome most commonly results from damage to the supramarginal gyrus or surrounding areas (see Fig. 2.1.).

The area most associated with writing ability is the angular gyrus, which is the posterior extension of Wernicke's area, and is situated at the junction of the temporal, parietal, and occipital lobes. Lesions which include the angular gyrus area cause Gerstmann's syndrome, consisting of dysgraphia, dyscalculia, right–left disorientation, and a peculiar deficit in recognition of body parts called finger agnosia.

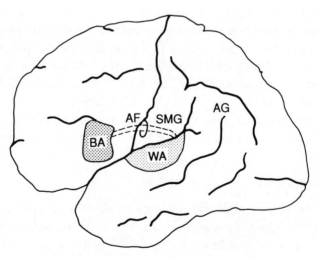

Fig. 2.1 Principal language areas (BA = Broca's area; WA = Wernicke's area; AF = arcuate fasciculus; SMG = supramarginal gyrus; AG = angular gyrus).

The minor hemisphere and language

The above statements concerning language dominance require some qualification, since not all aspects of language show such hemispheric specialization. It has become apparent from experimental studies of split-brain subjects (i.e. studies following corpus collosal section for intractable epilepsy) that, even in right-handers, the right hemisphere has a considerable capacity for understanding simple words, especially nouns, although it is unable to utilize the apparatus of speech for responding. This limited ability of the non-dominant hemisphere may explain some of the recovery seen even after devastating left hemisphere damage with resultant global aphasia. Also notable is the right hemisphere's role in some non-linguistic aspects of language expression and comprehension. Although the linguistic components—phonology, syntax, and semantics—convey the principal meaning of language (see below), there is in addition more subtle modulations which we use to imply attitude and emotion. These features have been termed **prosody**, which refers to the melody, pauses, intonation, stresses, and accents which enhance and enliven speech. Severely dysprosodic speech occurs with anterior left hemisphere damage. More subtle deficits in conveying and interpreting the emotion or affective components of language consistently accompany right-handed lesions—so-called 'emotional dysprosody'.

Neurolinguistics made simple

True aphasia results from the breakdown in the linguistic components of language. These can be divided into phonological, semantic (or lexical), and syntactic aspects.

Phonology

This is the term applied to the sound-pattern of human language. The smallest segment of spoken language is the phoneme, which is more or less the same as the sound represented by a single letter of alphabetic writing systems, such as the sounds represented by the letter 'k' in 'kiss' or the letter 'f' in 'fish'. Each language consists of a finite number of phonemes, which can be ordered to produce an almost infinite number of words. They can therefore be considered the building-blocks of language. Patients may be impaired in the ability to organize phonemes in sequence, which results in phonemic (or literal) paraphasias, which may be real-word approximations (SITTER for SISTER; STALE for SNAIL, etc.) or neologisms (FENCIL for PENCIL; POOT for SUIT; BORINGE for ORANGE). Phonemic decoding (necessary for distinguishing PEAR from BEAR, or FIT from BIT) is clearly critical for language comprehension. Both phonemic production and decoding depend on the superior temporal region.

Semantics

The term semantics denotes the referential meaning of words. The fact that we know the correct meanings of 'aunt', 'uncle', 'sister', etc., and that 'canary' refers to a small yellow bird, depends on normal semantics. Our store of words is sometimes called the 'mental lexicon'; but semantics refers to more than a simple store of word-forms; it encompasses our whole fund of knowledge of the world. This is discussed more fully under the heading of semantic memory (see p. 16). Breakdown within the semantic system results in a failure to understand the referential meaning of words, so that on naming or in spontaneous speech semantic paraphasias (ORANGE for APPLE, SISTER for BROTHER, etc.) are produced. Mere failure to access the correct word in the lexicon typically produces word-finding difficulty, with abrupt cut-offs in speech or circumlocutions ('it's that thin green vegetable that you eat with your fingers'). Comprehension clearly depends on the accurate assignment of meaning to heard words. A breakdown in this process impairs single-word comprehension. Again, the dominant temporal lobe plays a key role in lexico-semantic processes, although, as has already been mentioned, the right hemisphere appears to contain a limited but ineloquent lexicon.

Syntax

Words are strung together to form phrases or sentences in a complex way which obeys strict grammatical rules. The correct use of these non-substantive components of language—articles, prepositions, pronouns, adverbs, verb endings, etc.—is referred to as syntax. A reduction or complete loss of syntactic production, agrammatism, is found in patients with Broca's type aphasia. The production of sentences rich in these syntactic elements, but where they are incorrectly used, termed paragrammatism, is a feature of Wernicke's aphasia. Disorders of comprehension affecting predominately the syntactic aspects of language can also be demonstrated in some patients with damage to the inferior frontal lobe.

Table 2.1 Definitions and neural bases of language functions

Language function	Definition	Neural basis
Phonology	Production and comprehension of appropriately sequenced speech sounds (phonemes)	Left superior temporal lobe
Semantics	Assignment of meaning to words and production of linguistically appropriate individual words	Left temporal lobe (not well localized)
Syntax	Assembly of strings of words into sentences using pronouns, prepositions, tenses, etc.	Left anterior hemisphere
Prosody	(i) Fine tuning by intonation, stress, cadence, etc.	Left anterior hemisphere
	(ii) Emotional expression	Right hemisphere

Each of these components of language—phonology, syntax, and semantics—can be independently damaged. Furthermore, the deficit may involve input, output, or both. Since the neural circuits underlying these processes function in parallel and overlap anatomically, focal lesions invariably produce complex deficits. Many neurolinguists would argue that no two aphasia patients are exactly alike; but, luckily for clinicians, recognizable clinical syndromes usually emerge, at least after the phase of acute damage. It is worth emphasizing the point that the classical descriptions of the aphasic syndromes (Broca's, Wernicke's, and conduction aphasia, etc.) were based on chronic stable brain lesions. It is often difficult to apply this classification to acute stroke patients, the majority of whom have either a global aphasia or an atypical unclassifiable aphasia. Similarly, patients with language breakdown secondary to progressive degenerative brain disease, such as Alzheimer's or Pick's disease, do not develop classical aphasic syndromes. For these reasons, analysis of language disturbance is better considered in terms of the linguistic components outlined above.

The dual-route hypothesis of reading and writing

A similar linguistic analysis can be applied to disorders of reading and writing. In the case of writing, phonology becomes orthography (or spelling). In this respect, it is important to remember that the rules of English orthography are complex, with many unique exceptions. By knowing the rules of English pronunciation it is possible to read and spell many words correctly (HINT, GLINT, FLINT; GAVE, BRAVE, SAVE; etc.) and plausible non-words (NEG, GLEM, GORTH, etc.); but not words with irregular spelling-to-sound correspondence (for instance, PINT; HAVE; ISLAND). Clearly irregular words cannot be read *or* spelt correctly by applying spelling-to-sound rules, but rather must be pronounced or spelt by directly accessing word-specific knowledge about their phonology and orthography. The evidence from patients with acquired dyslexia supports the notion that there are two parallel systems for reading and writing; one utilizes sound-based route for reading and writing, and the other uses the more direct meaning route (see Fig. 2.2). These systems can break down independently, to produce different types of dyslexia and dysgraphia, which are described below.

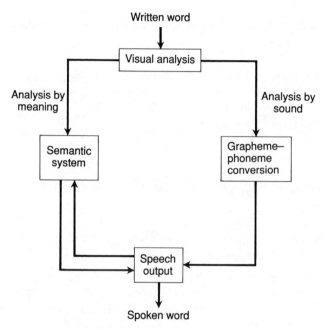

Fig. 2.2   Dual route model of reading.

Classifying aphasia syndromes

I have avoided the terms expressive and receptive aphasia, which, in my opinion, are misleading; virtually all aphasic patients have difficulty with language expression, although the linguistic processes underlying the deficit differ. Patients with left anterior lesions have a disturbance of language output, producing laborious and distorted speech. Posterior lesions produce a fluent language output, with phonemic and semantic paraphasic errors. Both patient groups have problems with 'expression'.

For the purpose of gross clinical diagnosis and clinico-anatomical correlation, four aspects of language should be considered (see Table 2.2).

Table 2.2 Classification of aphasic syndromes according to four parameters

Type of aphasia	Fluency	Repetition	Comprehension	Naming
Global	Non-fluent	+	+	+
Broca's	Non-fluent	+	−	+
Transcortical motor	Non-fluent	−	−	+
Wernicke's	Fluent	+	+	+
Transcortical sensory	Fluent	−	+	+
Conduction	Fluent	+	−	+
Anomic	Fluent	−	−	+

+ affected; − relatively spared.

1. *Fluent versus non-fluent:* This distinction divides aphasic syndromes into those related to damage anterior and posterior to the sylvian fissure. Non-fluent speech is slow and laboriously produced, with abnormal speech rhythm and melody, poor articulation, shortened phrase length, and often a preferential use of substantive words (especially nouns and some verbs). Non-fluent speech is invariably associated with lesions anterior to the sylvian fissure. Fluent speech, by contrast, is produced at a normal rate, with preserved speech rhythm and melody, good articulation, and normal phrase length. In fluent dysphasia the lesion is located posterior to the sylvian fissure, in or around Wernicke's area.

2. *Repetition:* When repetition is defective the lesion is in the peri-sylvian area, or so-called 'zone of language'. The latter is in the

territory of the middle cerebral artery, and includes both banks of the sylvian fissure, incorporating Broca's area anteriorly and Wernicke's area posteriorly—and the arcuate fasciculus between them. Where repetition is well preserved compared with spontaneous speech the lesion has spared these primary language areas, and is located cortically or subcortically outside the peri-sylvian region. Syndromes associated with sparing of repetition are termed transcortical—either transcoritcal motor or transcortical sensory.

3. *Comprehension:* Virtually all dysphasic patients will show some degree of comprehension deficit if tests of syntactic comprehension are used. However, for clinical purposes patients can be readily divided into those with obvious impairment of spoken language comprehension—invariably associated with a damaged superior temporal lobe (Wernicke's area)—and those in whom comprehension is spared.

4. *Naming:* The ability to name objects, or drawings of objects, is impaired in all aphasic patients to some degree. The type of errors, however, varies, as does the response to cueing, as will be described below.

Common aphasic syndromes: Broca's, Wernicke's Conduction, Transcortical, Anomic

For each of the more common aphasic syndromes I shall describe the nature of the spontaneous speech, performance on tests of naming, repetition, and comprehension, writing and reading, and their anatomical localization.

Broca's aphasia

In the fully developed syndrome, speech output has two principal characteristics—it is non-fluent and agrammatic, although these two features can dissociate. Typically, there is impairment of word initiation and phoneme selection. This results in slow, effortful, and laboured speech, which is distorted with frequent word approximations (phonemic paraphasias). Attempts at word or sentence repetition show the same features. The second major component of spontaneous speech is agrammatism. This is a simplification of grammatical form, with a notable reduction in function words (prepositions, articles, etc.). At its most severe, the patient is restricted to telegraphic utterances. It should be noted that this feature is present only in a minority of cases; most patients with Broca's aphasia manifest only a simplification or reduction in syntactic complexity rather than an absolute loss.

Naming on confrontation is impaired, but the patient often responds when a phonemic cue (the beginning sound of the word) is provided, and is able to choose the correct name from amongst a number of alternatives. Auditory comprehension, although typically preserved in ordinary conversation, may break down when it is studied by using syntactically complex commands. The written output of patients with Broca's aphasia mirrors their spoken language. It is characterized by mis-spellings, letter omissions, perseverations, and agrammatic sentences. Reading aloud is disturbed. On single-word reading, the syndrome of deep dyslexia (see p. 64) may occur, in which subjects make frequent semantic errors (SISTER FOR UNCLE; PARROT for CANARY, etc.), and are unable to read small function words, or unfamiliar, phonologically plausible non-words (CHOG, LAVE, GORTH).

Anatomical localization: The term Broca's aphasia has become more descriptive than anatomical. Neuroimaging studies have shown that lesions purely restricted to Broca's area (the inferior frontal lobe) produce a transient disturbance in speech output, not the other features of Broca's aphasia. The symptom complex of Broca's aphasia occurs after more extensive damage to the fronto-patietal region, corresponding to the area supplied by the superior branch of the middle cerebral artery. Moreover, the fully developed syndrome is rarely encountered in acute stroke patients, but evolves over time from a more global aphasic syndrome.

Wernicke's aphasia

In Wernicke's aphasia, spontaneous speech is fluent and paraphasic. In the acute stages speech output often consists of strings of phonemic and semantic paraphasias and their combinations, sometimes producing neologistic jargon. In contrast to Broca's aphasia, there is little effort in speaking, and no dysarthria. Indeed, in many cases there is an increased speech production rate, with a tendency to acceleration. Melody and intonation are preserved. It would, therefore, be impossible to detect Wernicke's aphasia in a patient speaking a language unfamiliar to the examiner. There is relative preservation of grammatical structure, but speech lacks information-conveying nouns and verbs ('Yes, I should say so, I mean, I'm a redax, no toxicat, that is to say . . ., you know what I mean', etc.). Often abnormal syntactic structures are produced; this is termed paragrammatism. Patients are usually unaware of their communication problem. Naming is severely impaired; patients often produce phonemic or semantic errors, but are not aided by phonemic cues, and are typically unable to select the correct name when offered a choice by the examiner.

Auditory comprehension is always impaired. In severe cases, patients are unable to point on command to common objects in an array (for example, 'point to the keys'); but simple body commands may be preserved. Linguistically, patients have difficulty with phoneme discrimination, and with assigning significance to perceived phonemes, i.e. matching words to their internal semantic representation.

The comprehension of written text is usually similar to auditory comprehension. However, some patients have superior reading ability, perhaps in association with relative sparing of more anteriorly placed parts of the superior temporal lobe. When writing, letters are well formed, but patients produce paraphasic, disjointed, and repetitive text, containing few nouns and verbs.

Anatomical localization: Unlike Broca's aphasia, Wernicke's aphasia correlates well with destruction of Wernicke's area. Right-handed patients with the full-blown syndrome of fluent, paraphasic, and paragrammatic speech and severe impairment of auditory comprehension almost invariably have suffered damage to the posterior superior temporal lobe of the left cerebral hemisphere. The extent of the comprehension deficit and the prognosis for recovery depends on the degree of damage to Wernicke's area.

Conduction aphasia

Named after damage to the main conducting tract (arcuate fasciculus) joining Broca's and Wernicke's areas, conduction aphasia is characterized by fluent but paraphasic speech. The paraphasias are mainly phonemic (for instance SITTER for SISTER; FENCIL for PENCIL). In contrast to Wernicke's aphasia, comprehension of speech and written material is much better. Repetition is highly abnormal; patients typically produce strings of phonemic approximations in an attempt to repeat a phrase, termed *conduit d'approche* (Roy Artery . . . Royit Artillery . . . Royot Artimery, etc.). Digit span is characteristically very limited. There is almost always anomia because of multiple phonemic paraphasic errors. Reading aloud parallels the performance of repetition; but comprehension of silent reading may be very good.

Anatomical localization: The traditional locus of pathology in conduction aphasia has been in the supramarginal gyrus, i.e. the gyrus lying above and around the posterior end of the sylvian fissure and the adjacent white matter tracts (see Fig. 2.1, p. 48), which thereby separates the temporal from the frontal language areas. Many exceptions to this classic localization have been reported, although most cases have involved lesions round the sylvian fissure. Conduction aphasia most often occurs at a stage of recovery from Wernicke's aphasia. When it occurs as an acute syndrome the prognosis for complete recovery is very good.

Transcortical aphasias

Early aphasiologists observed that some patients with aphasia retained competence at repeating language which they did not understand. They postulated the existence of a 'transcortical pathway' directly linking the so-called 'auditory language centre' and the 'verbal motor centre', thereby bypassing meaning. The term 'transcortical' has persisted, despite abandonment of the supporting theory, and is now used purely descriptively.

The features common to the transcortical dysphasias are preserved repetition and cortical or deep white matter damage at, or beyond, the periphery of the peri-sylvian language areas.

Transcortical motor aphasia (TMA) shares many similarities with Broca's aphasia: spontaneous language output is very sparse and dysarthric, but with few paraphasic errors. Sentence repetition is, by contrast, strikingly preserved, and comprehension of verbal and written language is very good. Written output parallels spoken output. Lesions responsible for TMA are located in the dominant frontal lobe anterior and superior to Broca's area. This is the type of aphasia typically seen with anterior cerebral artery infarction, and may follow a period of initial muteness. In these cases the critical lesion is in the supplementary motor area in the supero-medial parasagittal region of the frontal lobe. TMA may also occur in patients with focal lobar atrophy involving the frontal lobes (Pick's disease).

Transcortical sensory aphasia (TSA) is similar to Wernicke's aphasia, the language output being fluent but contaminated with semantic paraphasic errors. Comprehension is severely defective at the level of linking sound to meaning. Phonemic processing is, however, intact, and the patient is therefore able to repeat words and long sentences, but cannot extract meaning from language. Reading and writing are similar to those in Wernicke's aphasia. The site of the lesion is said to be in the border zone of the parieto-temporal junction, which therefore preserves the primary language areas, but disconnects them from posterior brain areas. A language syndrome akin to TSA occurs in advanced Alzheimer's disease and in patients with focal lobar atrophy affecting the temporal lobes (Pick's disease).

Anomic aphasia

Difficulty in word-finding on confrontational naming tasks is the rule in virtually all aphasic patients. Problems with word-access in free conversation, producing either abrupt cut-offs in mid sentence, circumlocutions, or paraphasic subsitutions, are also ubiquitous. Only when the severity of naming problems stands out above all other language deficits is the term anomic aphasia used. This is a common syndrome. It is a frequent residual deficit following recovery from one of the other types of aphasia, and is the characteristic language abnormality in the earlier stages of Alzheimer's disease. A space occupying lesion present anywhere in the dominant hemisphere may manifest as anomic aphasia.

Anomia is, therefore, the least useful localizing sign in aphasia. But the acute onset of pure anomic aphasia suggests a lesion in the left temporo-parietal area. When the injury extends to the angular gyrus, alexia and agraphia may appear.

Category-specific anomia is the term given to a deficit in naming items of a particular category. A well-documented form of this is colour anomia. Patients have a specific deficit in naming colours on confrontation or in pointing to colours when they are named by others (see p. 88). Other examples of category-specific anomias involve naming living things or non-living things. In the latter syndromes there is loss of general knowledge about the affected category, so that generating definitions, answering questions about semantic features, and comprehending on picture-pointing tests are also impaired. Since these deficits affect more than purely naming, they are more properly considered as disorders of semantic memory (see p. 17). Patients who have sustained temporal lobe damage from *Herpes simplex* virus encephalitis seem to be particularly vulnerable to category-specific semantic memory deficits.

It is worth noting at this point that the process of naming, although apparently simple and automatic in normal circumstances, depends upon a complex sequence of processes—visuo-perceptual, semantic, lexical, phonological, and articulatory—each of which may break down. Disorders of visuo-perceptual and semantic processing are considered more fully under the heading of visual agnosia (see p. 79).

Formal tests of language (see Appendix for details)

1. Spontaneous language elicited by complex picture description (for example the Beach scene illustrated in Chapter 4 and the Cookie jar theft picture from the Boston Aphasia Examination)

2. Naming to confrontation of the line-drawings graded in familiarity (for example the Boston Naming Test, Graded Naming Test)

3. Comprehension of increasingly syntactically complex commands (for example The Token Test)

4. Word–picture matching tests of single-word (semantic) comprehension (for example the Peabody Picture Vocabulary Test)

5. Aphasia batteries such as the Boston Diagnostic Aphasia Examination (BDAE), the Western Aphasia Battery, and the Porch Index of Communicative Ability (PICA) all provide a systematic and thorough evaluation of language abilities, but are time-consuming and not generally used in routine clinical neuropsychological practice.

Disorders of reading—the dyslexias

Disturbances of reading can be divided into two broad categories: (i) those in which there is a defect in the early visual components of decoding written script, the so-called **peripheral dyslexias**, and (ii) those in which there is a breakdown in the normal linguistic processes involved in deriving meaning from words, the **central dyslexias**.

Peripheral dyslexias: pure alexia; neglect dyslexia

Alexia without agraphia (pure alexia)

This rare syndrome has been important in establishing the concept of internal disconnection of cortical areas. In most cases there is an acute inability to comprehend any written material. By contrast, the patient recognizes words spelled aloud. Writing is preserved, but patients are unable to comprehend their own written output. With time, the ability to read individual letters often returns. When this happens, words are spelled aloud by the patients and recognized auditorily, so that they adopt a 'letter-by-letter' reading strategy. Because of this, there is a marked word-length effect, so that, unlike normals, patients with letter-by-letter reading are very slow at reading longer words. The syndrome is usually accompanied by right homonymous hemianopia. Defects in colour naming (with intact colour vision) or actual impairment of colour perception (achromatopsia) may also occur (see p. 88). This symptom complex usually accompanies infarction of the medial aspect of the left occipital lobe and the splenium of the corpus callosum, following occlusion of the left posterior cerebral artery (see Fig. 2.3). The proposed mechanism for alexia without agraphia is as follows: because of the right hemianopia patients cannot read in the right visual field. Words can be seen on the left side, and are therefore projected to the right hemisphere. However, the lesion in the splenium prevents transfer of the visual information from the right to the left side. The primary language areas are spared, but are disconnected from incoming visual information. The strategy adopted of identifying each individual letter is thought to occur initially in the right hemisphere, which then enables access to pronunciation in the left hemisphere.

Neglect dyslexia

In neglect dyslexia, which usually complicates right parietal lesions, there is failure to read correctly the left half of words (for example LAND is read for ISLAND; PEACH is read as BEACH, etc.). This syndrome is discussed more fully in the context of other hemineglect phenomena (see p. 74). Neglect dyslexia arising from a left hemisphere lesion and thereby affecting the right half of words is exceptionally rare and difficult to detect.

Central (linguistic) dyslexia: surface and deep dyslexias

Most aphasic patients have some disturbance of either reading aloud or of comprehension of text. Indeed, this is one of the most sensitive

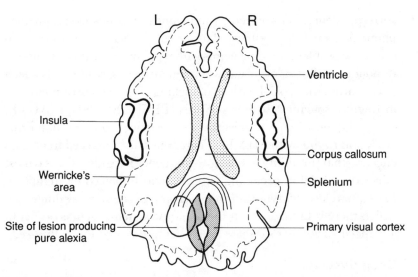

Fig. 2.3 Alexia without agraphia: lesion causes interrupton of information flow to the left-sided language areas from ipsilateral and contralateral visual areas (via splenium).

markers of language disturbance, and many patients who have otherwise recovered from acute aphasic syndromes find that they no longer derive pleasure from reading. In the aphasic syndromes, reading aloud usually parallels other oral language abilities. Broca's aphasics have particular difficulty reading grammatical morphemes (function words like OF and AT, and verb inflections like -ED) and make numerous errors, producing laboured and faltering oral reading. Their comprehension of complex text is usually poor. Most patients with moderate or severe Wernicke's aphasia are severely dyslexic, and make numerous paraphasic errors.

Two broad types of linguistically-based dyslexic syndrome can be distinguished on single-word reading (see Fig. 2.2).

Surface dyslexia

In this form of dyslexia, there is breakdown in the whole word (lexical) representations, so that reliance is placed on sub-word correspondences between letters and sounds (the so-called grapheme–phoneme conversion system). This use of the 'surface' features produces few problems reading words with regular sound-to-spelling correspondence. But errors occur when attempting to read words which deviate from the typical pattern of spelling-to-sound correspondence in English, so-called exception words (PINT, ISLAND, MAUVE, etc.). The most frequent mistake is to produce regularization error (PINT to rhyme with MINT). There is usually a marked frequency effect, so that the ability to read low-frequency irregular words is most affected. As well as occurring with posteriorly placed left temporo-parietal strokes, this syndrome may accompany dementing illnesses in which there is breakdown in the semantic system, such as occurs in advanced Alzheimer's disease and in temporal lobe Pick's disease.

Deep dyslexia

This syndrome is characterized by an inability to translate orthography directly to phonology, which means that patients with this disorder are required to read entirely via meaning, and are thus completely unable to read plausible non-words (NEG, GLEM, GORTH etc.). The cardinal symptom which is likely to bring attention to deep dyslexia is the semantic error: when trying to read single words aloud, the patient produces responses related in meaning (but not sound) to the target (for example, reading CANARY as PARROT; TULIP as CROCUS; SISTER as UNCLE, etc.). Visual errors are also common (for example, SWORD for WORDS, SCANDAL for SANDALS). There is usually great difficulty in reading small function words (IS, OF, AND, THE, etc.), and a relative impairment in reading abstract compared with concrete words. Most patients with deep dyslexia have suffered extensive left hemisphere damage. Opinions are divided as to whether the features of deep dyslexia result from the residual malfunctioning left hemisphere, or from the right hemisphere's attempt at reading. The latter gains support from the characteristics of right hemisphere reading in split-brain patients, which resemble in many ways the features of deep dyslexia.

Phonological dyslexia is a rare form of dyslexia that affects mainly the ability to read non-words.

Tests of reading ability (see Chapter 4 for details)

1. Text reading
2. Single-word reading using words with regular and exceptional spelling-to-sound correspondence, and plausible non-words
3. Single-letter identification

Disorders of writing—the dysgraphias

The production of well-formed and linguistically correct flowing script depends upon the integration of motor control, visuo-spatial and kinaesthetic function, and the symbolic aspects of the language system. It is not surprising, therefore, that writing abilities are fragile, and that brain dysfunction of very varied types produces dysgraphia. Three main varieties of writing disturbance can be identified.

Dyspraxic dysgraphia

Writing disturbance is said to have a dyspraxic quality if there is a disturbance in the smooth automatic production of written elements due to a breakdown in motor control. Letters may be inverted or reversed, and are often illegible. Copying is also abnormal. Oral spelling is preserved. Dyspraxic dysgraphia most often accompanies dominant parietal lobe damage, and features of ideomotor limb dyspraxia are usually present. Dominant frontal lobe lesions may occasionally produce pure dyspraxic dysgraphia.

Spatial or neglect dysgraphia

This disorder of writing usually accompanies non-dominant hemisphere lesions. It can be easily differentiated from the other

Table 2.3 Types of dyslexia and their localizations

Types of dyslexia	Localization
Peripheral dyslexias Preserved oral and written spelling, and ability to identify words spelt aloud	
1. Alexia without agraphia —letter-by-letter reading	Left medial occipital lobe
2. Neglect dyslexia —errors reading left-hand or initial part of words	Right hemisphere lesions
Central linguistic dyslexias Linguistically-based, invariably effect oral spelling	
1. Surface dyslexia —Breakdown of whole word (lexical) reading —Difficulty with irregularly spelt words —Phonologically plausible errors	Left temporo-parietal region and dementias
2. Deep dyslexia —Loss of sound-based (phonological) reading —Semantic errors —Difficulty with function and abstract words —Inability to read non-words	Extensive left hemisphere lesions

dysgraphias because of the invariable association with other visuo-spatial and perceptual abnormalities (spatial neglect, drawing problems, etc.), and by the characteristics of the writing: a wide left margin and a tendency to miss out, or mis-spell, the first few letters of individual words (RUSH for BRUSH; DOY for JOY, etc.).

Central (linguistic) dysgraphias: lexical (surface) and deep dysgraphia

These almost always accompany some degree of spoken language disturbance or dyslexia. The pattern of deficit tends to parallel the accompanying aphasia. Anteriorly placed dominant hemisphere lesions produce slow effortful writing which is poorly formed, with mis-spellings, omissions, reversals, and perseverations. Agrammatism may also be observed. Patients with Wernicke's aphasia may have preserved motor aspects of handwriting ability, but produce paraphasic errors and show word-finding impairments.

In keeping with the dual-route model of reading and writing previously discussed, two broad types of linguistic dysgraphia can be distinguished.

Lexical (surface) dysgraphia

The lexical (semantic) system uses whole-word retrieval by consulting internal memory stores of known spellings. This system is important for spelling familiar but orthographically irregular words (for example, CHOIR, PINT, ISLAND, NAIVE) and homophones (words with the same pronunciation but different spelling, for example ATE–EIGHT). Damage to this system produces a lexical agraphia characterized by particular problems in spelling irregular words and the production of error which are phonologically plausible (MENIS for MENACE, COFF for COUGH, etc.). This syndrome has been described in patients with lesions in rather diverse sites in the left temporo-parietal region. It is also a fairly consistent finding in patients with advanced Alzheimer's disease and with focal temporal lobe atrophy (Pick's disease) in whom there is a breakdown of the semantic system.

Phonological and deep dysgraphia

The alternative, phonological, spelling system uses sound–letter (phoneme–grapheme) rules. Disruption of this system produces phonological agraphia, in which patients are unable to spell unfamiliar words and non-words (for example VIB, CHOG, LAVE).

Deep dysgraphia results from more profound breakdown in the sound-based spelling route, with additional damage to the semantic system. As in deep dyslexia, semantic errors occur (SISTER for AUNT; SKY for SUN), and there is a strong effect of word class, in that those affected are better at spelling concrete than abstract words. Most patients with this syndrome have suffered extensive left hemisphere damage.

In the majority of patients with linguistically based agraphias, oral and written spelling are equally impaired. As a general rule, disturbed writing with spared oral spelling suggests a dyspraxic or neglect dysgraphia.

Tests of writing ability (see Chapter 4 for details)

1. Spontaneous writing of sentences

2. Writing words with regular and exceptional spelling-to-sound correspondence and plausible non-words

3. Copying words and single letters

Syndromes of calculating impairment

Acalculia, anarithmetria, spatial dyscalculia

Acalculia, a disturbance in the ability to comprehend or write numbers properly, is common in patients with aphasia; but rare instances where number and language abilities dissociate have been reported. The angular gyrus region in the left hemisphere appears important for numeracy. A separate disorder, **anarithmetria**, is characterized by the inability to perform number manipulations. Patients with this disorder correctly recognize and reproduce individual numbers and know their values, but cannot perform computations (addition, subtraction, etc.). This disorder is com-

Table 2.4 Types of dysgraphia and their localizations

Types of dysgraphia	Localization
Dyspraxic dysgraphia Oral spelling intact, defective copying	Dominant parietal or frontal lobe
Neglect dysgraphia Wide left margin or mis-spelling of initial part of words. Other neglect phenomena present.	Right hemisphere lesions
Central (linguistic) dysgraphias: written and oral spelling affected	
1. Lexical (surface) dysgraphia —breakdown of lexical route for spelling —difficult spelling irregular words —phonologically plausible errors	Left temporo-parietal region and dementias
2. Deep dysgraphia —breakdown of sound-based route for spelling —semantic errors —unable to spell non-words —better concrete than abstract spelling	Extensive left hemisphere damage
3. Phonological dysgraphia —as above, but without semantic errors	Unknown

mon in patients with dementia of Alzheimer type. A third cause of difficulty performing written calculations is so-called **spatial dyscalculia**. This syndrome, in which patients have difficulty aligning columns of figures and performing carrying tasks, complicates right hemisphere damage, and is invariably associated with other neglect phenomena (see p. 74).

Gerstmann's syndrome

This rare symptom complex is also referred to as the **angular gyrus syndrome**, because of the localization of the causative lesions. The features are:

1. Agraphia of the central (or linguistic) type.

2. Acalculia, producing difficulty with number reading, number writing, or calculations.

3. Right–left disorientation, by which is meant a disorder in demonstrating the correct hand (or other body part) to command.

4. Finger agnosia, a term applied to deficits ranging from the inability to name the fingers to inability to point or move a finger when its name is given. A more subtle indicator of this can be a difficulty in locating the fingers(s) touched by the examiner.

Since these features can occur in isolation or in any combination the usefulness of this syndrome in clinical practice is rather questionable.

Disorders of praxis—the apraxias

Apraxia is the inability to carry out complex motor acts despite intact motor and sensory systems and co-ordination, good comprehension, and full co-operation. The term 'apraxia' should be applied only to deficits with a motoric basis. Several unrelated disorders use the same term (dressing apraxia, construction apraxia, verbal apraxia of speech), but really deserve more accurate titles, and will not be considered in this section. Three main types of motor apraxia are recognized.

Table 2.5 Types of apraxia and their localizations

Types of apraxia	Localization
1. Ideomotor	Left parietal or frontal lobe
2. Orobuccal	Left inferior frontal lobe
3. Ideational	Corpus callosum; also found in dementia

Ideomotor apraxia

This disorder commonly accompanies aphasia. Patients are unable to carry out motor acts to command, but typically perform the same acts spontaneously. There is difficulty with the selection, sequencing, spatial orientation, and movements involved in gestures (waving, beckoning, etc.), and in demonstrating the use of imagined household items (for example, a toothbrush or comb) or tools. Imitation may improve performance, but does not correct the deficit.

In right-handed patients, almost all cases of apraxia are associated with left hemisphere lesions. The critical areas are the inferior parietal and pre-frontal areas. Such lesions may either destroy motor engrams (cortically stored movement patterns) or disconnect the flow of information necessary for initiating complex motor acts. Anterior callosal lesions can cause the inability of one limb—usually the left—to perform on command, even though the other limb performs normally.

Orobuccal (oral) apraxia

Patients with oral apraxia have difficulty performing learned, skilled movements of their face, lips, tongue, cheeks, larynx, and pharynx on command. For example, when they are asked to pretend to blow out a match, suck a straw, or blow a kiss, they make incorrect movements. The critical areas for lesions causing this deficit are the inferior frontal region and the insula. Thus oral apraxia commonly accompanies Broca's aphasia. Many of the speech-output deficits in Broca's aphasia may result from apraxia of speech (i.e. difficulty with articulation and phonation secondary to impaired motor programming). But occasionally Broca's aphasia and oral apraxia may occur in isolation.

Ideational apraxia

This term has been applied to the inability to carry out a complex sequence of co-ordinated movements, such as filling and lighting a pipe or making a cup of tea, although, in contrast to what happens in ideomotor apraxia, each separate component of the sequence can be successfully performed. However, it has also been used to describe the inability to use real objects (for example, a tooth-brush), even though the mimed use is retained. In either case, the deficit appears to be fairly rare. Ideational apraxia has been described in association with extensive left hemisphere and corpus callosal lesions, and in advanced Alzheimer's disease. In the latter group it is virtually impossible to unravel the contribution of apraxia from the confounding effects of poor language comprehension and diminished attention.

Damage to specialized right hemisphere functions

Deficits related to right hemisphere damage (in right-handed individuals) are much more difficult to detect than those caused by comparable dominant hemisphere damage. Often the deficits are subtle, and have not been noticed by the patient or observers. It is, therefore, arguably more important to assess any patient with suspected cognitive impairment carefully for these deficits, since aphasia and apraxia will usually be readily apparent.

It should also be noted that all the functions described in this section are only **relatively lateralized** to the right hemisphere:

spatial and visuo-perceptual skills are both bilaterally represented, but the hemisphere non-dominant for language is more specialized with aspect to these abilities. The deficities described in this section are more severe and long-lasting with right hemisphere damage, but virtually all of them can be found to lesser degrees with left-sided lesions.

Table 2.6 Deficits arising from right hemisphere damage

---

1. Neglect phenomena*
    Personal: Denial of hemiplegia (anosagnosia)
    Unconcern over deficit (anosodiaphoria)
    Neglect of grooming, shaving, etc.

    Motor and sensory: Hypokinesia
    Visual, auditory, and tactile neglect
    Sensory extinction to simultaneous bilateral stimulation

    Extrapersonal: Hemispatial neglect (e.g. drawings, line bisection, visual search)
    Neglect dyslexia and dysgraphia

2. Dressing apraxia*

3. Constructional apraxia*

4. Complex visuo-perceptual deficits*
    Object recognition (apperceptive visual agnosia)
    Face processing (prosopagnosia)

5. Prosodic components to language
    e.g. melody and intonation, especially emotional components

6. Vigilance/arousal, as part of attentional control (see Chapter 1)

---

* NB: These functions not very well lateralized, but deficits are more common and more severe with right hemisphere damage.

Unilateral neglect

There is substantial evidence that the right hemisphere in man is more important than the left for spatially-directed attention. The term 'attention' is applied rather broadly in neuropsychology to a number of different phenomena. I have used the qualifier 'spatially-directed' to separate this form of attention directed to personal and extra-personal space from the more general meaning of attention in the context of concentration/attention, which was discussed in Chapter 1. Deficits in spatially-directed attention produce unilateral neglect.

The term 'neglect' has been used to describe a complex of behavioural abnormalities. At its most profound, there is neglect of attention to extrapersonal and personal space. Patients behave as if one half—usually the left—of the universe has ceased to exist. If hemiplegic, they may deny any impairment, a phenomenon termed **anosagnosia**. They may even deny the existence of half their body, claiming that their left arm is someone else's. More frequently, patients admit that they have a neurological deficit, but appear unconcerned about it. This has been termed **anosodiaphoria**. Initially patients with neglect may ignore stimuli presented to the side contralateral to their lesion, whether the stimulus is visual, tactile, or auditory. Later, they become able to detect these stimuli, but when given simultaneous bilateral stimulation will fail to report the stimuli presented to the contralateral side. This phenomenon is called **extinction to double simultaneous stimulation**. It is most often observed in the visual and tactile modalities. Patients with severe unilateral neglect shave, groom, and dress only their right side, and even eat the food on the right half of the plate only. Failure to move their head and eyes to the side opposite to the lesion and motor akinesia of the contralateral limb may also be observed.

When asked to copy a drawing of an object such as a clock or house, patients often fail to draw the left side, and when writing they may leave a wide margin on the left or omit the initial part of the word (**neglect dysgraphia**). On reading, there may be omission of the beginning of the line or even the initial letters of a word (**neglect dyslexia**).

This full house of neglect phenomena may be seen acutely after extensive right hemisphere damage. More often, only part of the symptom complex occurs, and components of extrapersonal and personal neglect may dissociate.

In milder cases there is often no external manifestation, and only through specific testing (for example by drawing, cancellation, or bilateral simultaneous stimulation tests) will the impairment be detected. Recent work has indicated that a letter or star cancellation test may be the most sensitive means of detecting hemispatial neglect. For details of these tests see below.

Applied anatomy

Neglect is very common in the acute stages following damage to either the right or left cerebral hemisphere, but it is usually short-lived. Severe persistent unilateral neglect is found most often following damage to the right inferior parietal lobe and pre-frontal cortex. Homologous areas in the monkey receive inputs from the higher-order sensory association cortex, the thalamic nuclei, and parts of the limbic system (especially the cingulate cortex). Outputs go primarily to the frontal eye fields, the striatum and the superior colliculus. Thus the parietal lobe can be considered as a centre for integrating sensory experiences, motivational responses, and visual search mechanisms. Although apparently widely distributed, these diverse brain areas—parietal cortex, frontal lobe, cingulate gyrus, thalamus, and reticular system—are all intimately linked by reciprocal connections. Lesions of any one disrupt the mechanisms of spatially-directed attention, and may therefore produce neglect phenomena. Acute frontal lobe injury usually results in ipsilateral head and eye deviation, accompanied by visual and personal neglect phenomena. Lesions of the thalamus, the basal ganglia, or the cingulate gyrus may also cause unilateral neglect.

Mechanisms of neglect

Many patients with unilateral extrapersonal neglect have accompanying hemianopia, and it is tempting to attribute nelect to the visual loss. However, neglect may also be seen in patients with intact visual fields, and many patients with complete hemianopia are able to orientate and follow into their blind half-field, and furthermore do not show neglect phenomena on drawing or cancellation tasks.

One popular model proposed to explain the occurrence of neglect after right hemisphere lesions is as follows. Whereas the left hemisphere contains mechanisms which maintain attention to the contralateral (right) half of the sensory world, the right hemisphere contains the neural apparatus for attending to both sides of space. Thus lesions of the left hemisphere produce no substantial deficit, since the intact right hemisphere can take over the task of attending to the right side. Right hemisphere damage, on the other hand, will cause left unilateral neglect, since the intact hemisphere lacks the mechanisms for ipsilateral attention (see Fig. 2.4). To explain the phenomena of personal neglect, it has been proposed that the parietal lobe contains representations of the body with these same asymmetries.

However, it is clear that hemispatial neglect is not so easily explained. In a now famous experiment carried out in Milan, patients with neglect were asked to describe the cathedral square as if standing on the cathedral steps overlooking the square. They accurately described the features on the right side of the square, but omitted the details on the left. They were then asked to imagine that they were standing at the opposite end of the square, facing the cathedral. Now, they described all the features to their right (which had previously been omitted) and neglected those to their left (which had previously been included). This neglect of internal imagery has subsequently been reported in many neglect patients, and can be tested at the bedside by asking patients to imagine they are walking down a very familiar street and to describe all the

buildings they would pass. The basis for this type of representational neglect is unclear. It has been postulated that the right
hemisphere is responsible for constructing a central map of space
which is a direct analogue of sensory experience.

At present, there is no entirely satisfactory unitary hypothesis to
explain the diverse phenomena observed in neglect patients. It is
probable that both models of spatial attentional mechanisms and
internal representational models are in part correct.

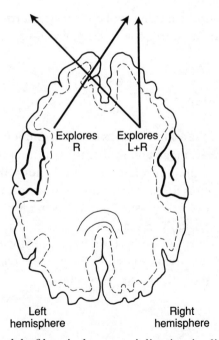

Fig. 2.4 A model of hemisphere specialization in directed attention
in which only a right-sided lesion will lead to unilateral visual
neglect.

Tests for unilateral neglect (see Chapter 4 and Appendix for details)

1. Spontaneous representational drawings (for example of bicycle, a house, etc.)

2. Copying of symmetrical drawings (for example of a two-headed daisy, a clock-face, etc.)

3. Line disection, in which the subject has to mark the half-way point on a number of lines of variable length

4. Letter or star cancellation—in these tests the subject is given piece of paper covered with randomly distributed letters or star or a mixture of both and is asked to cancel the target items (fo example, the small stars)

5. The Behavioural Inattention Test is a standardized battery fo detecting and measuring the severity of visuo-spatial neglect (se p. 197).

Dressing apraxia

A disturbance in the ability to dress is fairly common following foca right hemisphere damage and more diffuse brain injury. The term apraxia is, in fact, inappropriate, since it is not a motor disorder Instead, the deficit is in the orientation of body parts in relation t garments because of faulty visuo-spatial mechanisms. When there i a focal lesion, it is usually in the right posterior parietal area. Othe phenomena of right hemisphere damage are invariably present Patients with more advanced dementia or acute confusional state (delirium) may show the same problem.

Constructional ability

Impairment in the ability to copy a visually presented model b drawing or assembling blocks has been termed constructiona praxia. As with dressing apraxia, this bears no relationship to motor disorders. Apraxia is, therefore, a poor term.

To copy adequately a two-dimensional shape, such as a cube or star, requires normal visual acuity, the ability to analyse and perceive the elements of a drawing, and, finally, co-ordinated visuo-motor ability. Given the complex nature of the task, it is not surprising that deficits can arise with right- or left-sided cerebral damage. However, constructional apraxia is more common and more severe in lesions of the right hemisphere, especially if the parietal lobe is involved. There are also qualitative differences. Left-sided lesions lead to over-simplification in copying. Right-sided cases make gross alterations in the spatial arrangement, with so-called 'explosion' of the constituent parts.

Tests of constructional ability (see Chapter 4 and Appendix for details)

1. Copying three-dimensional shapes (for example, a cube) or the overlapping pentagons from the Mini-Mental State Examination (see p. 185)
2. Copying the Rey–Osterrieth Complex Figure.

Complex visuo-perceptual abilities—the agnosias

Although both hemispheres are involved in the processes of visual analysis, there is evidence for right hemisphere specialization. Patients with right-sided lesions have more substantial deficits on a range of visuo-perceptual tasks, including:

1. 'unusual views' tests, in which subjects are asked to match photographs of the same common objects photographed from conventional and from more unusual viewpoints, or to identify objects photographed from unusual viewpoints;
2. tests in which subjects are asked to identify items in overlapping line-drawings, or from partially degraded or fragmented images;

3. judgement of line orientation, which requires the subject t match a single test line to lines in a larger array (see p. 202); and

4. tasks requiring the analysis and matching of faces, often photographed from different angles and with different lighting conditions.

A battery of standardized tests for the detection of abnormalitie of this type, the Visual Object and Space Perception Batter (VOSP, see p. 220), is available, but is not suited to routine bedsid use.

Subtle deficits in perceptual processing are impossible to detect a the bedside; but severe disorders of visuo-perceptual processing may result in various forms of visual agnosia, which should b recognizable clinically.

Visual object agnosia

The term 'agnosia' can be roughly translated as 'non-recognition' Visual agnosia implies a disorder of recognition which cannot be attributed to general intellectual impairment, aphasia, or basi sensory dysfunction. A patient with visual object agnosia see objects, but fails to recognize what they are. Agnosias may be visual tactile, or auditory. Within a particular modality, agnosia can occur for different classes of stimuli such as colours, objects, or faces Often patients are agnosic for more than one class of items, and sometimes in more than one modality. However, pure disorders also occur. Since visual object and face agnosia are most common, have concentrated on these.

There are two principal types of object recognition disorder: one involves the earlier perceptual stage of object analysis; in the other there is a breakdown in the processes by which meaning is ascribed to visual percepts (see Fig. 2.5). These disorders have been termed 'apperceptive' and 'associative agnosia', after the work of Lissauer in the late nineteenth century.

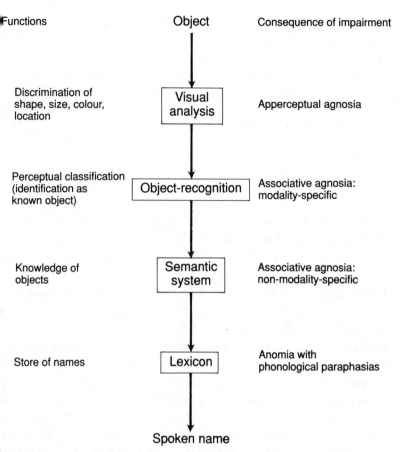

Fig. 2.5 A cognitive model of object recognition, understanding, and naming.

Apperceptive visual agnosia

Patients with this form of visual agnosia show preserved elementary visual faculties, such as acuity, brightness discrimination, and colour vision, but fail on more complex tasks involving object identification and naming. They are typically unable to copy shapes, or to discriminate in arrays two examples of the same object.

Table 2.7 The differentiating features of apperceptive agnosia and associative agnosia

	Basic visual processing	High-level perceptual analysis	Naming and identification	Semantic knowledge
Apperceptive agnosia	−	+	+	−
Associative agnosia	−	−	+	±*

* In some cases semantic knowledge is preserved, whereas others show a pervasive disorder of object knowledge.
+ impaired; − preserved

Visual fields may be normal; but most patients have defects on perimetry ranging from left hemianopia to marked tunnel vision. Despite being totally unable to identify visually presented objects, patients retain full knowledge about the unidentified items, and can name them by palpation or if given a verbal description. For instance, if shown a watch, patients with apperceptive agnosia would be unable to identify it as such, but if allowed to hold it would name it correctly. If asked to name the item 'worn on the right and used to tell the time' they would have no difficulty retrieving the word 'watch'. The neuropathology in apperceptive visual agnosia usually involves fairly widespread bilateral posterior occipito-parietal regions. Interestingly, carbon monoxide poisoning appears to have a particular aetiological role. Cases with bilateral posterior watershed strokes, penetrating head injury, and mercury poisoning have also been described. More restricted deficits in the identification of complex visual stimuli may occur with circumscribed right posterior parieto-occipital lesions.

Associative visual agnosia

This term has been applied rather broadly to patients with the inability to recognize visually presented objects despite apparently normal high-level perceptual processing. In classic cases the deficit is confined to the visual modality, while in others the deficit is more pervasive, and reflects a loss of stored semantic knowledge. The specific disorder of optic aphasia (see p. 84) is also sometimes included in this category.

Classic (modality-specific) associative agnosic patients have difficulty identifying or naming *visually* presented objects. Preservation of even high-level perceptual processing can be demonstrated by their normal copying of objects they cannot recognize, and by their ability to match pairs of such stimuli as the same or different. The traditional interpretation of this deficit considers the functional lesions to be one of accessing stored semantic knowledge from the visual modality, as a result of a disconnection in the flow of information (see Fig. 2.5). More recently it has been shown that high-level perceptual processes may not be entirely normal— patients are consistently better at recognizing real objects than photographs or line drawings, and the naming errors are invariably visual in nature. The site of pathology in such patients is variable: all have posterior quadrant damage, and in many it is bilateral; but cases with left unilateral posterior temporo-parietal lesions have also been documented.

In most cases of associative agnosia the deficit appears to be a more generalized semantic memory impairment. The defect in object recognition is, therefore, *not* limited to visual presentation. These patients demonstrate an inability to identify objects by any modality (for instance touch, or verbal description), as well as a loss of verbal knowledge which affects fine-grained (attributional) rather than broad category information. That is, they will be able to identify a picture as an animal, but unable to specify the type of animal. Likewise, on multiple-choice questions they will identify the word 'tiger' as the name of an animal, but make mistakes when asked about its size, habitat, ferocity, etc. A number of patients have been described in whom the loss of semantic knowledge is 'category-specific', for instance affecting living but not man-made things.

Such deficits are considered more fully in the section on semantic memory (see p. 16). The locus of damage in patients with deficits in semantic memory invariably includes the left temporal lobe. A degree of global semantic memory loss, resulting in features of associative agnosia, is present in patients with moderately advanced Alzheimer's disease, and to a more marked extent in patients with focal lobar atrophy of the temporal lobes (Pick's disease, see p. 39). Interestingly, in patients with 'category-specific' impairments, the cause is very often *Herpes simplex* virus encephalitis.

Optic aphasia

In this very rare syndrome, decribed by Freund in 1889, there is a disorder naming or verbally describing visually presented items. In contrast to what happens in visual agnosia, however, patients with optic aphasia can recognize items visually, as demonstrated by their accurate pantomiming of their use, even though they cannot access their names. The deficit is modality-specific, in that naming by tactile presentation and naming to description (for example, what do you call 'a large triangular musical instrument with many strings played by plucking?') are intact. Various explanations have been advanced to explain this strange syndrome. One influential account postulates a disconnection between stores of visual and verbal semantic knowledge. Thus object presentation activates intact visual knowledge, but verbal semantics cannot be assessed via this route; whereas, when one is given a verbal description, there is no difficulty with name access. Most cases are associated with right-sided visual field defects, achromatopsia, and/or alexia, since the site of damage is usually the left medial occipital region.

Tests for the detection and classification of visual object agnosias (see Chapter 4 for details)

1. Object naming (patients with visual agnosia produce visually and semantically-based errors)

2. Object description and miming of use

3. Copying of drawings

4. Naming to description (for example, what do you call the object 'worn on the wrist to tell the passage of time'?, etc.)

5. Ability to provide semantic information about unnamed items (for example, 'tell me everything you can about X')

6. Tactile naming

Balint's syndrome

This rare syndrome has three components: (i) psychic paralysis of gaze, that is to say an inability to direct voluntary eye movements to visual targets; (ii) optic ataxia, the inability to reach for, or point to, visual targets, also referred to as visual disorientation; and (iii) a visual attentional deficit in which only one stimulus at a time is apparently perceived, and even the attended stimulus may spontaneously slip from attention; this last feature is termed 'simultanagnosia'.

Patients complain of severe visual difficulties, and may appear to be functionally blind. When faced with arrays of items or complex pictures they appear to be able to attend to only one small area at a time, with a resultant inability to synthesize the parts into a whole. Despite this severe limitation in what they can see at one time, visual fields may be full when they are challenged with gross stimuli. But when asked to point to or touch the stimuli they make major errors in spatial localization.

The brain damage responsible is always bilateral, and includes the superior parieto-occipital region, damage to which interrupts the flow of spatial information from primary visual to parietal association areas. Cerebrovascular disease and prolonged hypotension leading to watershed infarction are the usual causes, although bilateral tumours may also result in the same syndrome.

Prosopagnosia

This term describes the inability to recognize familiar faces. While patients state that all faces are unfamiliar or unrecognizable, they are able to use cues such as voice, gait, or distinctive clothing to identify familiar people.

Following contemporary models of cognitive processing, face identification proceeds from a perceptual to a recognition stage, whereby faces are categorized as familiar, and then compared with stored representations of known faces before the appropriate name can be produced (see Fig. 2.6).

In prosopagnosia the deficit is at the categorization stage of this process, since these patients are able to describe and identify facial components (for example, beard, nose, etc.) and match faces in arrays containing examples of the same and different faces. In many cases they even retain the ability to perform complex visual matching tasks requiring the matching of faces taken under different lighting conditions and from different angles, although such tasks are usually performed slowly and laboriously. They also retain their knowledge of people they are unable to recognize, so that they may be unable to recognize a photograph of the Queen, but when given the name can produce appropriate factual information. Not surprisingly, prosopagnosics are invariably impaired at learning new faces.

The question of how selective the deficit is to face processing is controversial; most, if not all, cases have problems with fine-grained identification such as types of flower, breeds of dog, makes of car, etc., leading some authorities to speculate that prosopagnosia is a defect in distinguishing items within categories containing many confusable exemplars.

Prosopagnosia is most commonly associated with bilateral inferior occipito-temporal lesions, but occasional (non-autopsied) cases with purely right-sided lesions have been reported. Field defects are usually present, and many patients have additional deficits such as achromatopsia or pure alexia.

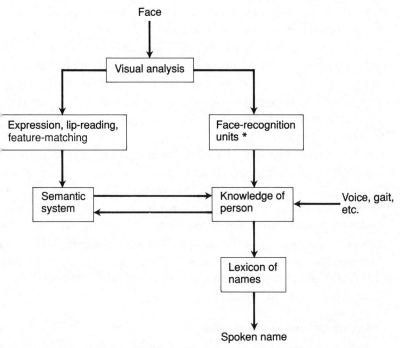

Fig. 2.6 A cognitive model of face recognition. Face recognition units function as a memory-store of known faces. A lesion at this level (*) causes prosopagnosia.

Tests of face-processing (see Chapter 4 for details)

1. Naming and description of photographs of familiar persons

2. Matching of photographs in arrays containing examples of the same face (sometimes taken from different angles or in different lighting conditions) amongst other faces.

Achromatopsia, colour agnosia, and colour anomia

Achromatopsia is an acquired disorder of colour perception characterized by a loss of ability to discriminate between colours. It may occur in isolation from other defects in object or form perception. It is usually symptomatic; patients complain that everything appears washed out, or 'like black and white TV'. It may affect part or the whole of the visual field. The critical site of pathology is the medial occipito-temporal region. Pure alexia (alexia without agraphia, see p. 61) and achromatopsia in the right hemifield often occur together after left posterior cerebral artery territory infarction.

In contrast, patients with **colour agnosia** are able to perceive and distinguish between colours, but are impaired on tasks requiring the retrieval of colour information (for example, 'What colour is a banana?'). A specific disorder in colour naming with preservation of colour perception and of colour knowledge has also been reported under the heading of **colour anomia.** The latter syndrome may also be associated with alexia and right-hemianopia and is attributed to a disconnection of the left hemisphere language centre from visual information.

Tests of colour processing

1. Colour discrimination (i.e. distinguishing colours and matching examples of the same colour in arrays)

2. Colour naming (i.e. producing the correct colour name when shown coloured objects or colour samples)

3. Colour knowledge (for example 'What colour is a banana?' etc.)

3. Cognitive history-taking and tips on physical examination

The patient interview

The importance of establishing an accurate and detailed account of the patient's cognitive problems and their evolution cannot be over-emphasized. It is also essential to obtain an independent account from the patient's spouse/partner or, if necessary, another family member or close friend. This applies particularly in the area of memory disorders and behavioural/personality change, where the patient is frequently unaware of his or her deficit. By the end of the interview it should be possible to formulate a fairly accurate provisional diagnosis, or at least to delineate the areas of cognitive function requiring particular attention on examination.

Suggested structure of interview

1. Introduce yourself and other staff present.

2. Outline the plan of the interview and examination.

3. Interview the patient, preferably alone, explaining that you wish to hear about his or her symptoms and problems. If the informant remains present, tell him or her that you would like to talk first to the patient without the 'help' of the relative. Make sure that you do talk to the patient alone at some stage; there may be important confidential facts that he or she wishes to impart, or personal questions that would be inappropriate with others present.

4. Interview the informant alone.

5. Physical and cognitive examination. Again, it is essential to do

this with the patient alone to gain a true picture and to avoid
embarrassing the patient and his or her family.

For the full assessment of a new patient I allow an hour, which is
often not long enough for a full cognitive assessment, but should
allow a working diagnosis to be reached. Further neuropsychological testing will often be necessary.

Beginning

Before embarking upon the history of the presenting complaint, try
to establish a rapport with the patient by asking a few general, non-
confrontational questions about the patient's background, such as
place of birth, schooling, past jobs, family, hobbies, and interests.
Even at this stage valuable information is gained. Clearly, if the
patient is unable to engage in sensible conversation and answer
simple questions accurately and coherently, then further attempt
to take a history from the patient in person will be impossible and
pointless. In this situation the informant will be vital in providing
information about the current problems and background.

Reason for referral

Does the patient know why he or she has been referred to the clinic
or why he or she is in hospital? In ordinary medical practice, we
usually assume that patients are fully aware of the reasons for their
referral. In patients suffering from cognitive deficit this is not
always the case. It is revealing to enquire why they think they are
being seen. Questions need to be phrased sensitively to avoid
insulting or patronizing the patient, but can usually be achieved
with something along these lines: 'I like to ask all of my patients to
tell me why *they* think they have been referred to see me.' It is
surprising how often patients think that they are being seen about a
skin complaint or bad hearing!

Open-ended questioning

Continue the interview by asking general 'open-ended', rather than
leading, questions. This provides the best opportunity to obtain a

non-biased narrative account of the patients' problems. Some suggestions are:

• Tell me how your problems first started.

• What are your main areas of difficulty at present?

• What impact has this had on your work, family, hobbies, etc.?

• What are the activities that you are having difficulty with?

Try to record in the hospital notes phrases used by the patient verbatim. These are often much more meaningful and useful to future doctors than statements such as 'complaining of memory difficulties' or 'six years progressive dementia'.

Direct questions

In all cases the narrative account obtained by open-eded questions needs to be supplemented by questions designed to probe specific domains of cognitive function. In this way, an overall pattern of abilities in each area can be built up. Valuable additional information will be obtained by questioning the patient's relatives. Indeed, in more impaired patients this supplementary information is by far the most important. A check-list for use with patients and informants is given below.

Check-list for interviewing patients and informants

1. Memory
   • anterograde: recall of new episodic information in day-to-day life (for example, recalling messages and conversation, family news, TV programmes, etc.)
   • retrograde: past personal and public event memory

   • semantic: vocabulary, names and general factual knowledge (history, geography, politics, etc.)

2. Language
- output: word-finding, grammar, word-errors (paraphasias)
- comprehension of words and grammar
- reading
- writing: spelling and motor components

3. Numerical skills
- handling money, shopping, dealing with bills

4. Visuo-spatial skills
- dressing
- constructional abilities
- spatial orientation and route-finding

5. Neglect phenomena
- neglect of extrapersonal space
- bodily neglect

6. Visual perception
- recognition and identification of people
- object and colour identification

7. Hallucinations
- visual, auditory, tactile, olfactory

8. Personality change and social conduct, including eating habits, sexual behaviour

9. Thinking and problem-solving abilities

10. Depression
- mood
- energy, concentration
- biological features (appetite, sleeping)

1. Memory

The complaint 'memory difficulty' is used in a variety of ways by patients and relatives. Try to establish if the patient is referring to memory for names of specific people, places, and things, in which case the deficit is one of semantic memory. Alternatively, and more commonly, the term is applied to memory for personally experienced events or recently acquired information (messages, news items, shopping, conversations, etc.), in which case the deficit is one of episodic (event-based) memory. Poor memory may also be the principal complaint in patients with attention deficits and in patients with depression.

The other useful distinction, clinically and neuropsychologically, is between memory for newly encountered information (anterograde memory) and memory for past events (retrograde memory). Usually these are affected in parallel, and to a roughly equivalent degree, for instance in Korsakoff's syndrome and Alzheimer's disease. However, dissociations may occur; after closed head injury there is severe anterograde amnesia and limited retrograde; with selective damage to particular parts of the limbic system (for instance the hippocampus) fairly pure anterograde memory loss may occur.

Confabulation refers to the tendency to produce erroneous material on being questioned about past events. Confabulations may occasionally be grandiose and delusional, but more commonly consist of misordering and fusion of true past memories.

Reminder: Throughout this book I avoid (wherever possible) the confusing terminology of short-term and long-term memory. In experimental psychology, short-term refers to the very limited capacity store, lasting only seconds as measured by digit span. Alternative names for this short duration system are immediate or working memory. By contrast, clinicians and the general public usually refer to short-term memory as that assessed by name and address recall after 5 or 10 minutes (see p. 7 for a fuller discussion). Whenever I use 'short-term' it is in the neuropsychological sense.

Suggested areas of enquiry

Anterograde: Ability to remember new information, such a messages, telephone conversations, news stories, and importan personal material, such as family events. Does the patient need to use lists? Has he or she become repetitive? Does he or she frequently lose things while at home?

Retrograde: recall of past personal events such as holidays operations, jobs, and past homes. Recall of public and news items.

Semantic: names of people, places, and things. Vocabulary and factual knowledge. Deterioration in this domain often manifests a. difficulty with word-finding and naming, and in understanding the meaning of less common words.

2. Language

When questioning patients and their relatives about language problems it is useful to consider language in terms of production and comprehension.

Language production

- Is the patient as fluent and articulate as normal?

- Has there been a deterioration in grammar?

- Is there a misuse of words (paraphasias)? Most patients with aphasia produce incorrect or distorted words in spontaneous speech. The occurrence of semantic (for example, SISTER for BROTHER, APPLE for ORANGE) and phonemic (SITTER for SISTER) paraphasias may be noted by relatives.

- Is word-finding difficulty apparent? A degree of anomia specially for less common words, is more or less a universal accompaniment of aphasia, and is frequent from the early stages in dementia of Alzheimer type.

Language comprehension   Disorders of language comprehension often affect grammar (or syntax). This is often first apparent when trying to follow complex instructions and keeping track of group conversations. Using the telephone is particularly difficult for patients with any degree of comprehension deficit, because all the usual gestural and contextual cues to meaning are absent. In patients with temporal lobe damage or progressive degenerative diseases the understanding of individual words is also affected.

Reading Can the patient still read fluently with comprehension and pleasure? A reduction in leisure reading is a subtle indicator of mild dyslexia; but memory difficulties may obviously also complicate interpretation of this symptom. In dominant hemisphere injury, reading usually parallels spoken language; but in occasional cases pure alexia may occur. The rare, but well recognized, combination of alexia with preserved writing ability is a distinct and localizing syndrome, almost invariably associated with right hemianopia, and often with disorders of colour perception and verbal memory problems.

Writing If a history of writing difficulty is elicited, try to distinguish between breakdowns in spelling or in the motoric control of writing. In the latter, termed apraxic agraphia, oral spelling is preserved. Remember, most people write very little other than shopping-lists and postcards. Agraphia is, therefore, usually underestimated by relatives and patients.

Note: disorders of reading and writing do not always denote dominant hemisphere pathology. In neglect dyslexia patients may fail to read one side—usually the left side—of the page or individual words. Likewise, in neglect dysgraphia one portion of the page or word is omitted. Consider these syndromes if other aspects of spoken language are normal.

3. Numerical skills

Difficulty with manipulating numbers often manifests as inability to use money, and hence to shop alone. Ask also about management of household accounts.

4. Visuo-spatial skills

In contrast to language and memory disorders, which are usually clearly apparent to close observers, deficits in visuo-spatial ability may be clinically silent. It is, therefore, particularly important to make specific enquiries about potential symptomatology.

Dressing ability Impairment in the ability to dress oneself, so-called dressing apraxia, usually reflects a complex visuo-spatial deficit rather than a true apraxic (i.e. motor-based) problem. The act of putting on a shirt requires alignment of body parts and mental rotation, which depend upon the non-dominant hemisphere. Thus this type of dressing disorder usually occurs in the context of focal right posterior parietal lesions. Patients with frontal brain damage may show a different disorder of dressing, which consists of a mis-sequencing of garments, and results in wearing underpants on top of trousers, etc.

Constructional deficits These are rarely evident without formal testing. Occasionally patients with particular skills or professions (architects, model builders, etc.) may complain of difficulty drawing or in three-dimensional constructions, suggesting right parietal damage. It is always worth asking about hobbies. A specific decline in practical abilities such as DIY or drawing may also suggest right-sided pathology.

Spatial orientation Topographical disorientation, that is to say getting lost in familiar surroundings, is a common accompaniment of moderately advanced dementia. It may also indicate focal right hemisphere pathology. It may be due to poor spatial memory or to failure to recognize landmarks.

5. Neglect phenomena

Neglect of space Patients with focal right hemisphere lesions often fail to respond to stimuli in the opposite half of extrapersonal space. This may manifest as a failure to talk to visitors on the left side of the bed, a tendency to ignore food on the left half of the plate constantly bumping into objects and door-jambs on the neglected side, or even failing to read the left half of the page.

Bodily neglect   In its most profound form, patients deny the presence of hemiplegia despite evidence to the contrary. The term 'anosagnosia' applies to this phenomenon. Less dramatic versions, consisting of a tendency to ignore or under-use one side, are more frequent.

5. Visual perception

Misidentification   Patients with disorders of visual processing may think that faces on the television are actually in the room. Misidentification of familiar faces may also occur, and is common in delirium, when other illusions and hallucinatory experiences are often present. In the Capgras syndrome patients are convinced that a close relative (usually a spouse) has been replaced by an imposter who looks identical to their spouse. This rare syndrome occurs in dementia and in schizophrenic disorders.

Agnosia   There are a number of fairly rare syndromes involving the inability to identify faces, colours, or objects despite normal basic perceptual processes. In prosopagnosia, patients are unable to recognize faces belonging to friends, acquaintances, or famous people. However, they can identify these people correctly from voice, dress, or gait. A failure to recognize people by any sensory modality suggests a deifict of semantic memory. In some forms of object agnosia, subjects fail to recognize objects by sight, but can still identify the same objects by touch. Achromatopsia denotes a loss of colour vision with preserved acuity and object identification. Suggestions of useful screening questions are:

• Does he or she ever confuse you or other family members with someone else?

• Have you noticed any problems in recognizing familiar faces?

- Has he or she had difficulty in identifying everyday objects, or used things inappropriately?

- Have you noticed any problems with colour vision?

7. Hallucinations

In neurological patients visual and olfactory hallucinations are commoner than those in the auditory modality. Fairly often there is also at least partial insight. A particular form of visual hallucination, which involves seeing well-formed, and often remarkably realistic, images of animals, faces, and often children, is common in patients with advanced Parkinson's disease, when it is usually secondary to dopaminergic medication. It has been termed peduncular hallucinosis, since it was originally described in association with acute vascular lesions of the cerebral peduncles in the mid-brain. Formed visual hallucinations in the absence of cognitive impairment are known as the **Charles Bonnet syndrome**. Most patients with this disorder have poor eyesight. Vivid hallucinations are common in acute confusional states, when tactile hallucinations of crawling or itching may also occur. Olfactory and gustatory hallucinations are invariably fleeting, and may occur as part of the phenomena of complex partial seizures originating from the medial temporal lobe.

A sensitive way of enquiring about such phenomena is to say something like the following: 'Patients with various kinds of neurological disorder sometimes have unusual experiences when they see, hear, or smell things which may not be there. Have you had anything like that?'

When talking to relatives you should ask specifically whether the patient has ever seemed to be seeing or hearing things, or talking to non-existent people.

8. Personality change and social conduct

It is difficult to overlook major deficits in memory and language even with unstructured history taking, and visuo-spatial disorder hould be readily detected by a few simple pen-and-paper tests. Disorders associated with frontal lobe damage or disease, by contrast, are easily overlooked, and it is in these domains that nformant interview is extremely important.

Typical personality changes associated with frontal lobe dysfunction consist of apathy or adynamism, lack of concern about oneself and others, often with childish, egocentric behaviour, inability to empathize, and lack of inhibition, with a tendency to react mpulsively. A lack of spontaneity, with little initiation of conversation and activity, poor motivation, inattentiveness, and distractibility is common. Restlessness and constant pacing or wandering may occur. Not infrequently patients are aggressive toward family members. In advanced cases, relatives may note a deterioration in eating, grooming, and toileting habits. A tendency o bawdiness, such as telling inappropriate 'dirty' jokes and a general decline in manners, is commonly observed.

With bilateral temporal lobe damage, patients may develop features of the Kluver–Bucy syndrome, consisting of a tendency to eat indiscriminately, sometimes including inedible items (cigarette-ends, soap, etc.), without satiety, increased sexual drive, and emotional blunting and passivity.

. Thinking and problem-solving

Having covered each of the specific areas of cognitive function—language, memory, etc.—there remain the higher-order adaptive functions, which co-ordinate and integrate overall intellectual activities. Disorders of these higher-order or executive functions cause a general dimming of intellect, problems with mental flexibility, abstraction, and creative thought. Sequencing and planning are often severely impaired, leading to dropping off in performance at work or in household tasks and hobbies (DIY, gardening, bridge-playing, etc.).

Perseverative behaviour may be noticed. Poor judgement and an inability to modify behaviour according to changing situations are also commonly reported. Appreciation of jokes and puns also depends on complex abstracting ability, and so is frequently affected.

10. Depression

Atypical depressive illness is undoubtedly the commonest treatable disorder in patients presenting to a memory disorder clinic. As a general rule, complaints of poor memory and concentration should make you consider an affective illness—most patients with true memory impairment are relatively unaware of a deficit. Besides obvious questions about depressed mood, the following are useful lines of enquiry:

1. lack of pleasure from life (anhedonia);
2. preoccupation with pessimistic thoughts about the past and future;
3. loss of interest in the family, home, and hobbies;
4. poor concentration;
5. reduced energy; and
6. biological features, such as weight loss, anorexia, early morning wakening, and diurnal variation of mood.

The informant interview

The general format of the informant interview should follow that used with the patient. General open-ended questions should be used first, followed by directed questions to cover each area of cognitive function. Establishing the evolution, pattern, and impact of the deficits is the overall aim.

What were the first observed problems?

In the dementias this is particularly important, because in their end-stages all degenerative diseases tend to produce an indistinguishable picture. The earliest-noted deficit is, therefore, of important diagnostic value. For instance, if there is an insidious decline in anterograde memory, with preservation of personality and social behaviour, then the diagnosis is almost certainly Alzheimer's disease. Early change in personality and social conduct points to frontal lobe disease. Word-finding difficulty or speech hesitancy localizes the process to the dominant hemisphere. Spatial disorientation or dressing apraxia as the predominant problem alerts one to the right hemisphere, and so on.

Was the onset acute, insidious, or stuttering?

The mode of onset of cognitive problems is very important. Delirium is always abrupt in onset, and often fluctuating in its course. If an apparent dementing syndrome has an acute or subacute onset over days or weeks then a depressive pseudodementia should be suspected. The rate of progression is also helpful diagnostically: Alzheimer's disease progresses insidiously, multi-infarct dementia typically has a step-wise course, cortical Lewy body disease is associated with marked fluctuating disease, and Jakob–Creutzfeldt disease progresses extremely rapidly.

Situation-based problems

Instead of sticking to questions purely about individual cognitive domains it is often illuminating to enquire about particular difficulties in various everyday settings, such as:

- at work;

- in cooking and general housework;

- when driving;

- in using money and paying bills;

- in gardening and other hobbies;

- in social encounters with family and friends; and

- in grooming, toileting, and eating habits.

Impact on the family and personal relationships

Assessment of the impact of any cognitive change on the family is clearly very important. This also gives the opportunity to enquire about sexual activity. Contrary to the views of the young, sexual intercourse does not stop at forty, or even necessarily at seventy. Most spouses dealing with difficult and embarrassing changes in sexual behaviour will value your interest in this sensitive area.

Family history

It is inadequate to record in the medical notes 'Family History—nil relevant'. This is best exemplified by apparently *de novo* cases of Huntington's disease in which a family history is frequently said to be 'negative'. Detailed probing about the family background invariably reveals important clues, such as an uncle who committed suicide, a grandfather who died at a young age in a mental hospital, etc.

Besides noting the age, state of health, and cause of death of first-degree relatives, preferably in the form of a family tree, you should ask specifically about any family history of neurological or psychiatric illness. As most patients have no idea what constitutes illness in these areas, ask specifically about:

- senile dementia

- memory loss

- Alzheimer's disease

- Parkinson's disease

- epilepsy

- strokes

- mental breakdowns

- depression
- suicide.

Also enquire whether any family members have ever needed to see a psychiatrist.

Past medical history

Of particular importance in assessing cognitively impaired patients are the following:

1. significant head injury, i.e. injury associated with post-traumatic amnesia of more than one hour, neurosurgical procedures, skull fracture, or post-traumatic seizures;

2. epilepsy of any type;

3. previous CNS infections, either meningitis or encephalitis; and

4. psychiatric illness.

Alcohol intake

Opinions as to a reasonable level of alcohol intake vary considerably. Women are undoubtedly more susceptible to alcohol-mediated complications than men. The working party of the Royal College of Physicians recommend 'safe levels' of up to 21 units/week for men and 14 units/week for women. The same report suggests that 'hazardous' levels are 21–49 units/week for men and 14–35 units/week for women. 'Dangerous' levels are above these limits. Try to record the average weekly intake in numbers of units per week. One unit is equivalent to half a pint of beer, one glass of wine, or a measure of spirits. People often underestimate the extent of their alcohol intake, and it is often very useful to go through the last week on a day-to-day basis, adding up everything the patient can recall drinking. An independent assessment of alcohol intake should always be sought from the patient's spouse.

Tips on physical examination

It is not appropriate to describe here the complete neurological examination which should obviously be performed on all patients presenting with cognitive disorders. I shall concentrate instead on a few additional, and perhaps less commonly known, signs which are useful in the detection of focal cerebral abnormalities.

Cranial nerve signs

Smell: I myself do not test smell routinely. However, it should always be tested in the following circumstances: past history of head injury; dementia, especially of frontal lobe type; complaints of poor taste or smell; and the presence of visual symptoms or signs (suggesting subfrontal pathology).

Vision: As well as testing acuity (in each eye) and pupillary responses and fields, remember to examine for visual extinction or neglect in every patient. Visual extinction is the consistent tendency to ignore stimuli in one half field (or, rarely, one quadrant) when both sides are simultaneously stimulated by finger wiggling. The visual fields must first be shown to be intact when using single stimuli. Visual extinction is always pathological, and implies damage to the opposite posterior parieto-occipital area. Although included in the category of neglect phenomena it occurs commonly with right and left-sided brain damage. This is a good time to test for optic ataxia (visual disorientation) by asking the patient to touch your fingers whilst wiggling them in each quadrant with the patient fixating ahead. Whilst looking at the eyes also remember to observe for Kayser–Fleischer rings. These brown pigmented rings or crescents are best seen with the patient looking down whilst illuminated with a torch from the side, and are pathognomonic of Wilson's disease.

Eye movements: Abnormalities are most often missed because of too-rapid examination and a failure to test vertical eye movements. Gaze should be sustained in each of the primary positions, i.e. horizontal right and left, vertical up and down. As well as following (pursuit) movements, testing should include rapid voluntary side-to-side and vertical (saccadic) movements. These may be selectively disrupted in basal ganglia disorders (for example Huntington's disease). A severe and selective deficit in vertical eye movements occurs in progressive supranuclear palsy (Steele–Richardson–Olzewski syndrome), and also following upper brain-stem and thalamic strokes.

Frontal release signs

A large number of primitive frontal signs have been described. These are released from normal inhibition in the presence of frontal lobe damage or disease. Their interpetation is difficult, because some occur in a high proportion of the normal elderly, and they rapidly fatigue on testing. In descending order of usefulness they consist of:

1. Grasping. This is practically always pathological below the age of eighty. To elicit, lightly stroke your hand across the patient's palm whilst distracting the patient with casual conversation. A positive response consists of involuntary grasping, which can be fairly subtle. The patient does not have to grasp your hand like a vice for it to be abnormal!

2. Pouting. Ask the patient to close his or her eyes lightly. Place a spatula in the mid-point of his or her lips in the vertical plane. Warn the patient that you will tap the spatula firmly, but not too hard. A positive response consists of puckering of the lips towards the stick, as if to blow a kiss. This may be normal above the age of seventy.

3. Glabellar tap. With the patient sitting, tap gently and repetitively with the index finger in the mid-line between the eyebrows, keeping the rest of your hand out of view. Normal

subjects blink in response to the first two or three taps only
Continued blinking after five or more taps is considered positive
Many of the normal elderly have a positive glabellar tap.

4. *Palmo-mental response.* This is the least meaningful of the fronta
release signs. It is elicited by stroking the thenar eminence with ar
orange stick or a similar implement, and observing the contra
lateral mental muscle, which is situated on the chin. A positive
response consists of the contraction of this muscle.

Motor system

Postural arm drift: This is tested by asking the patient to maintain a
static position of the outstretched arms in the horizontal position
with the eyes closed. Downwards and usually inwards drift of the
arm is a frequent sign of contralateral hemisphere disease, and may
be found in the absence of any other motor signs. Observation of the
hands and fingers in this position is also very useful for detecting
involuntary choreiform or dystonic movements.

Involuntary movements: These are best observed when taking the
history. Chorea is often overlooked, and attributed to fidgetiness. If
there is any doubt about their presence, ask the patient to lie still on
the bed with the eyes gently closed. Also watch when the patient is
walking; this often exacerbates chorea, producing characteristic
finger-flicking movements, and may also bring out dystonic limb-
posturing.

Sensory system

Astereognosis This is a form of tactile agnosia in which the patient is
unable to recognize objects despite normal sensation, co-ordination, and motor function. Deficits are associated with contralateral
parietal lesions. It occurs equally with right- and left-sided damage.

Graphathesia The inability to recognize letters or numbers traced
on the palm or finger tips is also associated with damage to the
contralateral somatosensory parietal cortex. A few practice

numbers should be drawn for the patient with the eyes open, making sure that the numbers traced out are orientated towards the patient.

Sensory inattention This denotes a failure to appreciate a stimulus when a similar stimulus is applied simultaneously on the opposite side. For instance, patients can register when their right hands are touched, but when both sides are simultaneously touched they report only the left-sided stimulation. This method is often called double simultaneous stimulation. It occurs frequently with right and left parietal lesions.

Gait and balance

No neurological examination is complete without watching the patient rise from a seated position and walk twenty paces or so. Impairment in the initial stages, with the 'glued to the floor' sign, is characteristic of gait apraxia associated with normal pressure hydrocephalus. Small rapid festination, with a hunched posture and lack of arm swing, characterizes Parkinson's disease. Particular difficulty with turning or changing direction is a common accompaniment of Parkinson's disease and other degenerative extra-pyramidal disorders (such as progressive supranuclear palsy). The choreiform movements of Huntington's disease are frequently exacerbated by walking. Visual neglect may be apparent if the patient consistently bumps into objects to one side.

The 'stork' manoeuvre If the patient can balance on one leg with arms folded across his or her chest and eyes open then any significant disorder of balance and practically any lower limb pyramidal weakness can be excluded.

4. Testing cognitive function at the bedside

The general schema followed is that already outlined in Chapter 1. The first part of the examination assesses distributed cognitive functions; deficits in these indicate damage to particular brain systems, but *not* to focal areas of one hemisphere. The second part of the assessment deals with more localized functions, divided into those associated with the dominant (i.e. the left side, in right-handers) and non-dominant hemispheres.

At the end of the chapter there is a suggested minimum assessment protocol which can be used as a check-list; but supplementary testing is needed if deficits in specific areas are detected. The basic protocol takes approximately 15–20 minutes to administer.

Cognitive assessment should always follow history taking, because invaluable information is gained from the patient and informant which guides the examination. For instance, even minor degrees of aphasia should be apparent from history taking, and will lead the examiner to assess language function thoroughly.

General observations

Mood and motivation are essential to all mental functions. The degree of co-operation, the ability to sustain effort, and the amount of encouragement required to complete a task are all observable aspects of motivation. A disturbance in motivation is described as 'apathy', and if it is extreme the term 'abulia' is used.

Behaviour during the examination should be noted. Does the patient interact appropriately? Frontally damaged patients are often inappropriately jocular, or make puerile or obscene comments. Patients with acute confusional states (delirium) show either increased or decreased psychomotor activity. In the former state, patients are restless, voluble, noisy, fidgety, and distractable. In the latter, hypo-alert variant of delirium, patients are quiet, speak little, and drift easily off to sleep if unstimulated.

Orientation and attention

Alertness	Level of wakefulness and reactivity	
Orientation	• Time	Day of week Time of day Month Year
	• Place	Building Town County Country
	• Person	Name Age Date of birth
Attention/concentration	Serial subtraction of 7s Months of year backwards Days of week backwards Digit span forwards and backwards	

Alertness

Record the level of wakefulness of the patient. It is hopeless to attempt a detailed cognitive assessment in a drowsy patient. A common-sense description such as 'awake and fully co-operative', 'co-operative but sleepy, with a tendency to doze off if unstimulated', are much better than vague, undefined terms such as 'obtunded' or 'stuporose'.

Orientation

This is conventionally divided into time, place, and person Of these, the first is the most important and clinically helpful.

1. *Time* Time orientation should include the time of day, the day of the week, the month, and the year. Date orientation is extremely unreliable, since many normal subjects do not know the date. Also include a question such as 'How long have you been in hospital?' This is often helpful, because mildly disorientated patients frequently over- or underestimate the passage of time thinking that they have been in hospital for days when, in fact they were admitted only that morning.

Disorientation in time is common in patients with acute confusional states (delirium) due to metabolic disorders or diffuse brain injury. It is also seen in patients with moderate to severe (but not mild) dementia, and in the amnesic syndrome.

Note: many patients with clinically significant memory impairment remain well orientated in time. Orientation in time should not, therefore, be taken to exclude a significant memory disorder

2. *Place* I usually use a question something like, 'What is the name of this building?' It is surprising how often patients are unaware that they are in hospital, a fact that is easily overlooked if the examiner simply asks the name of the hospital. Orientation in place is less sensitive than time orientation to attentional and memory deficits.

3. *Person* It is rare for patients to be unable to tell you their names. Even very confused or demented subjects do not usually show this deficit. But it is a characteristic feature of psychogenic (hysterical) amnesia. Aphasic patients may also be unable to access their own names, but when given a choice, such as 'Is your name Frank, John, or Harry?', can usually pick out the correct name. Patients with aphasia are frequently misdiagnosed as confused because they are unable either to comprehend the

uestion or to produce the correct answer. This error should be voided if the patient is engaged in casual conversation before lunging into formal cognitive assessment. Also included as part of erson orientation are age and date of birth.

ttention/concentration

bility to sustain attention and keep track of ongoing events can e assessed in a number of ways, including digit span, serial ubtraction of 7s, spelling of familiar words backwards (for nstance WORLD—DLROW), and recitation of the days of the veek or the months of the year in reverse order. Of these, I favour he last. Many normal elderly subjects make errors of serial ubtraction, as do patients with focal left hemisphere damage. The nonths of the year are an overlearnt sequence, familiar to veryone. The ability to recite these in reverse order is, therefore, a ood measure of sustained attention. Patients should be fast and rrorless at this simple test. If the patient is unable to do this, try he days of the week backwards instead.

Digit span, especially reverse digit span, is also a good measure of ttentional processes, and a useful adjunct to the measures above. 'he ability to repeat a string of digits has little, if anything, to do vith the processes involved in laying down and retrieving new pisodic (event) memories. Digit repetition depends upon short-erm (working) memory, which in turn depends upon frontal xecutive and phonological processes (see p. 7). Reduction in digit pan is a feature of impaired attention, as found in acute onfusional states or moderate to severe dementia, and may also ccur in patients with focal left hemisphere lesions. Patients with phasia frequently have a reduced digit span.

Note: patients with the amnesic syndrome (for example, orsakoff's disease), who may be totally unable to lay down any ew episodic memories, have a normal digit span.

Digit span is tested by asking the patient to repeat a progres-ively lengthening string of digits. It is usual to start with three igits. Two trials are given at any level. If subjects pass on the first

or on the second trial, then the next-length sequence is adminis
tered. Digit span is the highest level at which the patient passe
either trial. The number should be read by the examiner at one pe
second—without clustering, which aids repetition: you only hav
to think of the usual way in which we recall telephone numbers

Forward digit span: example

6—2—7   correct
8—3—6   not administered
1—7—4—9   incorrect
7—2—5—1   correct
4—9—3—1—6   incorrect
3—8—4—7—9   incorrect

Forward span = 4 (impaired)

Exactly the same technique is employed on reverse digit span
however, here the patient is required to repeat the numbers i
reverse order. It may be necessary to give some patients severa
demonstrations at two digits. Normal digit span is 6 ± 1, depend
ing upon age and general intellectual abilities. Thus an intelligen
young adult would be expected to have a forward span of at leas
6. In the elderly, or those of low intellectual ability, 5 can b
considered normal. Reverse span is usually one less than forwar
span (see p. 200 for further details).

Memory

Anterograde verbal • Name and address recall
• Incidental recall of earlier conversation
journey to hospital, events on ward, etc
• Formal tests: story and word-list recall

Anterograde non-verbal	• Route learning
	• Face memory
	• Formal tests: Rey–Osterrieth Complex Figure Test, Recognition Memory Test (faces)
Retrograde	• Famous events, for example:
	Recent sporting events
	General elections
	Gulf War
	Russian coup
	Hillsborough Stadium disaster
	Herald of Free Enterprise disaster
	Falklands War
	Watergate affair
	Assassination of Kennedy
	Suez Crisis, etc.
	• Remote personal (autobiographical) memory

As has been previously discussed in greater detail (see p. 5), there are many sub-components to memory. To recap, in psychology, short-term memory applies to the system of working memory responsible for the immediate recall of small amounts of verbal or spatial information (tested at the bedside by digit span or immediate recall of a name and address), which bears little relationship to other aspects of clinically important memory. What we normally think of as memory—the capacity to learn and recall personally experienced events such as a meeting yesterday or last year's holiday—comes under the heading of episodic memory.

In clinical terms, episodic memory function is best considered as anterograde (i.e. the ability to learn new information) and retrograde (i.e. the recall of old information). This distinction is

particularly useful since different pathological processes ma
differentially affect one or other of these components. Semanti
memory describes our permanent store of knowledge about thing
in the world, as well as about words and their meanings.

Anterograde verbal memory

An informal, but often very revealing, impression of memory ca
be gained by asking patients to recall the details of very recen
events, such as their journey to hospital, their last meal, or event
on the ward. As a naturalistic test of such incident memory,
frequently employ the following technique: at the beginning of th
interview, in the course of our general conversation, I find a topi
of interest, such as the patient's family or a recent holiday, and tel
the patient something about my own family or holiday. Then late
I ask the patient to recall these facts.

Name and address recall: Have the patient repeat a name anc
address three times to ensure that it has been attended to anc
processed. Since repetition is within the span of short-term
(working) memory, this is a measure of general attentiona
processes rather than of memory proper. After five or ten minute
(the actual time is not critical) ask the patient to recall the nam
and address. It should be noted that this is a very crude measure
Total failure, or recall of one or two elements, is clearly abnorma
at any age. Completely correct recall shows that the patient doe
not have a *major* amnesic deficit, although many patients shown t
have a significant memory deficit on formal testing score perfectl
on this simple task. Intermediate results are always more difficul
to interpret. Clinical intuition is important. If informants are
concerned about a patient's memory, even if the defect is no
obvious on simple testing, then formal neuropsychological evalu
ation is required.

Formal assessment: For those interested, and who do not have
access to professional neuropsychological assessment, I woulc
recommend two measures: story recall and word-list learning
Both are quick and relatively foolproof. Furthermore, there are

ood normative data to guide interpretation. Several versions of
tories for recall exist, all of which derive originally from the
Wechsler Memory Scale. There are numerous word-list learning
asks. One of the most widely used is the Rey Auditory Verbal
Learning Test. Examples of both are given in the Appendix. For a
more thorough evaluation of memory abilities, the Rivermead
Behavioural Memory Test is an excellent assessment instrument
see p. 214).

Anterograde non-verbal memory

n the vast majority of patients with memory disorders, non-
verbal memory parallels verbal memory. However, damage to the
on-dominant—usually right—medial temporal lobe structures
may cause a selective non-verbal memory problem, such as a
problem with learning faces, geometrical figures, or spatial
ocations. Patients with early Alzheimer's disease are also very
ensitive to tests of non-verbal memory. Unfortunately there is no
asily administered bedside test of non-verbal memory. Spatial
earning can be tested by walking a route around the ward or
linic with the patient, and then asking him or her to repeat this
oute alone. *Ad hoc* tests of face memory can be made fairly easily
sing photographs from magazines of non-famous faces. The
Rey–Osterrieth Complex Figure Test provides very good inform-
tion on non-verbal memory. The subject is first asked to copy the
igure (which is obviously a test of visuo-spatial skills), and then,
fter a delay of 30 to 45 minutes, without being forewarned, the
ubject is asked to reproduce the figure from memory. Normative
ata is available, and is given in the Appendix.

The Recognition Memory Test is a valuable standardized test
f verbal and non-verbal recognition memory. In the face memory
ubtest subjects are shown 50 faces, each for three seconds, and
sked to make a value judgement as to whether they find the face
leasant or not. After finishing this part of the test, they are then
iven 50 pairs of faces, each containing one of the previously
ncountered faces, and asked to say which they have seen before.

Normals perform surprisingly well on this test, and good normative data are available. The Rivermead Behavioural Memory Test also contains subtests which assess picture (object) recognition and recall of a route around the room (see p. 214).

Retrograde memory

Assessment of retrograde or remote memory is impressionistic at best, but a reasonable overall picture can be achieved by systematic questioning about a range of past events from the preceding months, years, and decades. Interpretation must be tempered by the patient's likely baseline performance. For instance, elderly women are unlikely to know in detail about recent sporting events, and many normal subjects' grasp of political events is extremely sketchy! Recall is harder than recognition, so start with open questions, such as 'Can you tell me about any recent news items?' or, 'What important events have been in the news lately?' Amnesics often have a rough idea, so it is important to probe for specific details. It is useful to ask about a standard list of famous events, examples of which are given above. In virtually all patients with retrograde memory impairment there is a temporal gradient. That is to say they are much better at more distant events, and become progressively more impaired the nearer you get to the present. Patients with diencephalic amnesia (for example Korsakoff's syndrome) and Alzheimer's disease have a very extensive but graded remote memory impairment. In pure hippocampal damage the retrograde loss is typically much more limited—a year or two at most (see p. 14).

The other domain of remote memory is personal or autobiographical memory. An impression of the patient's capacity in this area is best formed during history taking. Can the patient accurately relate, and in the correct chronological sequence, events and details of his or her own life? The best formal test of remote personal memory is the Autobiographical Memory Interview (see Appendix).

Frontal executive functions

Initiation

- Verbal fluency tests:
  Letter fluency (F, A, S)
  Category fluency (Animals, Fruit,
    Vegetables)
  Supermarket fluency test

Abstraction

- Proverb interpretation
  e.g. 'One swallow doesn't make a
    summer'
  'Still waters run deep'
  'A bird in the hand is worth two in
    the bush'

- Similarities test
  e.g. 'apple and banana'
  'coat and dress'
  'poem and statue'
  'table and chair'
  'praise and punishment'

- Formal test: Cognitive Estimates Test
  (see Appendix)

Response-inhibition and set-shifting

- Alternating sequences
- Go–no-go
- Motor sequencing tests (Luria three-
  step and alternating hand movements)
- Formal tests: Wisconsin Card-Sorting
  Test and Trail Making Test (see
  Appendix)

The history obtained from an informant and general clinical observation of the patient's behaviour are more important than formal bedside testing for the overall assessment of the higher-order or executive functions. However, there are a number of measures which can be helpful in confirming clinical impressions.

Initiation: verbal fluency tests

The generation of words beginning with a specified letter, or from a common semantic category (for example animals, fruit, etc.) depends on the co-ordinated activity of two main cerebral areas— the frontal lobes, which generate retrieval strategies, and the temporal lobes, where the basic information is stored. Therefore, in the absence of aphasia (or, more particularly, of anomia), verbal fluency is a good test of frontal lobe function. In the standard version of the letter fluency test, patients are asked to generate as many words as possible, excluding names of people or places, in one minute. The most commonly used letters are F, A, and S. Normal young subjects should produce at least 15 words for each letter. A total for FAS of less than 30 words is abnormal; but some allowance should be made for age and background intellect.

In category fluency tasks, subjects are asked to generate as many examplars as possible from semantic categories such as animals, fruit, vegetables, etc. For the category animals, normal young subjects produce more than 20 items in a minute; 15 is a low average, and 10 is definitely impaired. Performance drops with age, and for the very elderly 10 may be just about acceptable (see Appendix).

As well as absolute numbers on both tasks, a note should be made of the number of perseverative responses. Normals do not perseverate. Patients with severe amnesia may produce perseverative errors; but in general they are a feature of frontal lobe disease or dysfunction of frontal lobe connections (for example Huntington's and Parkinson's diseases).

A related and clinically useful task is the Supermarket Fluency Test. In this, subjects are asked to list all the things that can be bought in a supermarket. Normal subjects systematically search various subcategories (dairy produce, fresh fruit, etc.), giving a few examples of each. On this test around 22 items is average, and 15 or below is impaired. Patients with frontal dysfunction show poor organization strategies and perseverative responses. In Alzheimer's disease, the patients attempt to search various categories, but produce few exemplars.

Abstraction: proverbs, similarities, and cognitive estimates

Some impression of abstract conceptualization can be gained from proverb interpretation and the similarities test. Suggestions of proverbs for administration are given earlier. Concrete interpretation, with an inability to make analogies, characterizes the performance of patients with frontal-lobe damage. For instance, 'one swallow doesn't make a summer' is usually interpreted as referring to the number of birds you need to see before summer has started. Interpretation of proverbs is highly dependent upon educational level and cultural background. Concrete responses may also be given by patients with schizophrenia.

The similarities test involves asking subjects in what way two conceptually linked items are alike, starting with simple pairs such as 'apple and banana' and 'table and chair', and progressing to more abstract pairs such as 'poem and statue' and 'praise and punishment'. The normal response is to form an abstract category (for example fruit, furniture, works of art). Patients with frontal deficits and dementia make very concrete interpretations (for example, table and chair: 'you sit at one to eat from the other' or 'both have legs') and often continue to do so despite being asked to think of other ways in which the items are alike.

Another useful test of conceptualization is the Cognitive Estimates Test, in which patients are asked a range of questions which require common-sense judgement to answer. Examples are 'How fast do horses gallop?', 'What is the height of the Post Office

Tower?', 'What is the height of an average Englishwoman?' and 'How many camels are there in Holland?'. Frontal patients give bizarre and illogical answers to these questions. The full test is given in the Appendix.

Response-inhibition and set-shifting

The ability to shift from one cognitive set to another, and to inhibit inappropriate responses, cannot be easily tested at the bedside. The best formal test of set-shifting is the Wisconsin Card Sorting Test which also involves problem-solving and hypothesis-testing. In this test the subject has to sort cards containing geometric forms which differ in number, shape and colour. Having deduced the correct sorting dimension, the subject is then required to shift to another dimension (for example, from colour to shape) on a number of occasions. Patients with frontal lesions are unable to shift from one sorting criterion to another, and make perseverative errors. See the Appendix for a fuller description.

The alternating sequences test provides a measure of this ability but is insensitive except in patients with gross deficits. The examiner produces a short sequence of alternating square and triangular shapes (see Fig. 4.1). The patient is asked to copy the sequence, and then to continue the same pattern until the end of the page. Many patients with frontal lobe deficits repeat one of the shapes rather than continuing to alternate the pair.

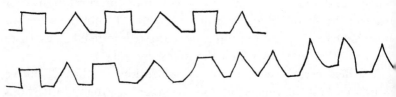

Fig. 4.1 An example of a frontal patient's copy of an alternating sequence.

Go–No-Go test   Response-inhibition can be tested using this paradigm. The patient is asked to place a hand on the table and to raise one finger in response to a single tap, while holding still in response to two taps. The examiner taps on the undersurface of the table to avoid giving visual cues. Patients with frontal deficits cannot inhibit raising one finger in response to the 'no-go' signal. Again, this is a relatively insensitive test, so that any abnormality is highly pathological.

Trail making   The Trail Making Test is a reasonably good quantitative measure of attention-shifting and response-inhibition. On Part A, the patient must draw a line connecting randomly arranged numbers in numerical sequence (1—2—3, and so on). On Part B, the numbers are intermixed with letters, and the test is to draw a line connecting numbers and letters in an alternating sequence so that the connecting line goes from 1 to A to 2 to B to 3, and so on. Performance is influenced by intelligence and age. Age norms are available. An example of the test and normative data are given in the Appendix.

Motor sequencing: the Luria three-step Test and the Alternating Hand Movements Test   Deficits in sequencing complex motor movements are associated particularly with left frontal lesions. A number of tasks can be used, of which the 'Luria three-step' and alternating hand movements tests are most helpful. In the former the examiner demonstrates the series of hand movements—fist, edge, palm—five times without verbal clues, and then asks the subject to repeat the sequence (see Fig. 4.2). Patients with frontal deficits are unable to reproduce the movements, even if given specific verbal clues.

In the Alternating Hand Movements Test the examiner again demonstrates the movement. The examiner starts with arms outstretched, one hand with fingers extended and the other with clenched fist. Then the hand positions are reversed by alternately opening and closing each hand in a rhythmical sequence (see Fig. 4.3).

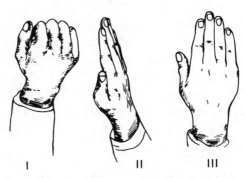

Fig. 4.2 Luria three-step Test: the sequence of hand positions (fist—edge—palm) is shown. Figure taken from *Higher cortical functions in man* by A. R. Luria. © 1966, 1979 by Aleksandr Romanovich Luria. Reproduced by permission of Basic Books, a division of Harper Collins Publishers Inc.

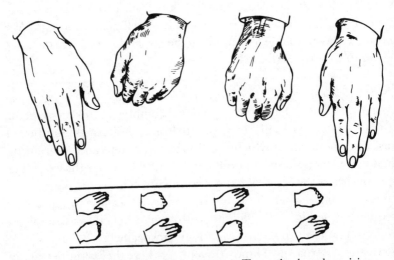

Fig. 4.3 Alternating Hand Movements Test: the hand positions (above) and the sequence of movements to demonstrate to the patient (below) are shown. Figure taken from *Higher cortical functions in man* by A. R. Luria. © 1966, 1979 by Aleksandr Romanovich Luria. Reproduced by permission of Basic Books, a division of Harper Collins Publishers Inc.

DOMINANT (LEFT) HEMISPHERE FUNCTION

Language

1. Spontaneous speech during conversation and picture description
   - Articulation
   - Fluency—phrase length
   - Grammatical form
   - Paraphasic errors
   - Word-finding
   - Melodic line (prosody)

2. Naming
   - Overall ability
   - Error types
   - Benefit from cueing with initial sound

3. Comprehension
   - Conversational understanding
   - Pointing to command:
     Single-word (semantic)
     Sentence (syntactic)
     Conceptual

4. Repetition
   - Words and sentences

5. Reading aloud and comprehension; if defective analyse the following:
   - Letter identification
   - Type of errors
   - Effects of regularity
   - Non-word reading

6. Writing
   - Spontaneous sentence composition

- Writing to dictation
- Oral spelling (if deficit is found in written spelling)

Calculation
- Number-reading and writing
- Arithmetic operations

Praxis
- Buccofacial
- Limb gestures $\Big\}$ command and imitation
- Object use

Language

Spontaneous speech

The analysis of spontaneous speech is the most important aspect of language examination for the classification of aphasia. This should be done after listening to several minutes of spontaneous conversation and after asking the patient to describe a complex scene such as the one shown on p. 148. However, it should be noted that this analysis is much more readily applied to aphasia resulting from strokes and other focal lesions than to the aphasia seen in patient with degenerative brain disease. Deficits can be considered under the following headings.

1. Articulation: are the words well-formed and articulated, or laborious and distorted? Disturbances of phonetic aspects of language often accompany anteriorly placed or deep left-hemisphere lesions.

2. Fluency: does the patient produce normal-length phrases between pauses? This should be disentangled with word-finding difficulty. Many patients with otherwise fluent aphasia have word-finding problems which break up their speech, but they are capable to producing occasional long phrases (5 or more words). Patients with non-fluent speech have a consistently low rate of production in

erms of words per minute, and produce short phrases. Phrase
ength should, therefore, by judged only after listening to several
ninutes of speech.

3. Syntactic (grammatical) form: does the patient produce speech
vhich obeys the rules of his or her native language? Agrammatic
peech is simplified, lacks grammatical words (pronouns, preposi-
ions, etc.) and contains errors of tense. Agrammatism correlates
losely with non-fluent language.

4. Paraphasic errors: are word-substitution errors present? These
nay be sound-based (phonemic paraphasias) such as SITTER for
ISTER, or FEN for PEN. Or they may be meaning-based
semantic paraphasias), as are JUG for GLASS and APPLE for
)RANGE. Severely paraphasic speech may contain non-words
neologisms), and in its most profound form produces jargon
phasia. Neologisms also occur in schizophrenic speech, but there
hey tend to be bizarre words used consistently, rather than with
ariable phonetic blends that characterize aphasia.

5. Word-finding: does the patient's speech have pauses followed
y circumlocutions (for instance, 'the thing you write on paper
vith') or clichés such as 'thingy' or 'whatsit'?

6. Melodic line (prosody): does the patient's speech have a normal
ntonation and stress, with a pattern of rising and falling pitch?
)isturbances in prosody often accompany poor articulation and
educed fluency. Patients with laboured and awkward speech
utput are unable to maintain a melodic contour. Disturbances of
motional prosody (i.e. of inflection, tone, and pitch used to express
motional states) may occur in right hemisphere damage.

Naming

The ability to name objects or pictures is impaired in virtually all
phasic patients, and is probably the best index of overall severity.
A range of items of varying similarity should be used, since aphasics,
n common with normal subjects, show a marked frequency effect.
That is to say, they are much more likely to show errors when
naming low frequency (less familiar) objects. This can be assessed

using everyday items and parts of objects. Watch and pen are high
frequency items; winder, buckle, and nib are low frequency items.
The type of error which occurs is also helpful diagnostically.
Patients with anterior (Broca's type) aphasia typically produce the
initial sound of a word, and are helped by phonemic cueing.
Conduction aphasias produce multiple phonemic errors (TELOP
TELE, TELEPHONT for TELEPHONE). Semantic paraphasia
(for example CLOCK for WATCH, APPLE for ORANGE) are
frequent in Wernick's aphasia, sufferers from which may produce
totally neologistic utterances. Semantic errors also characterize the
anomia of Alzheimer's disease. It should be remembered that
accurate identification of visually presented objects also depend
upon intact perceptual processes; the occurrence of visually-based
naming errors and difficulty in visual identification in the absence
of other language deficits should suggest a visual agnosia (see p. 79).
There are several easily administered formal tests of naming ability,
including the Graded Naming Test and the Boston Naming Test
(see Appendix).

Comprehension

It is common to overestimate the comprehension abilities of aphasi
patients on the basis of their understanding of unstructure
conversation. In free conversation there are gestural, facial, an
prosodic (tone-of-voice) cues. Thus, fluent aphasics can ofte
respond appropriately to opening conversational gambits ('How
are you today?'), depite profound comprehension problems. Body
part commands may also be very misleading; responses to axia
commands such as 'Close your eyes', 'Open your mouth', an
'Stand up' are commonly preserved. The reason for this preserva
tion is obscure.

On the other hand, testing comprehension with difficult three
part commands (for example, 'Touch your left ear with your righ
index finger and then touch my hand') lead to erroneou
underestimation of the comprehensional abilities, since these com
mands are not only grammatically complex, but also overloa

hort-term (working) memory capacity, and require right–left nderstanding.

Comprehension is best tested by asking the patient to point first n response to single words, then in response to sentences of ncreasing complexity, and then finally in response to conceptually-ased questions or instructions.

1. *Single-word comprehension:* using everyday objects carried in our pocket (for example, a coin, a pen, a watch, keys, etc.) and ems in the ward or clinic (for example, a bed, a chair, a desk, owers, etc.) ask the patient to point to each in turn. Remember to se a spectrum of items of differing familiarity and parts of objects, ince comprehension is always affected by this variable; severe phasics may be able to point to the common but not the less ommon ones.

2. *Sentence (syntactic) comprehension—'The Pen–Watch–Keys test':* .gain this can be easily performed using an array of three common bjects from your pocket. Having established that the patient can nderstand the name of these items, test comprehension using a ange of syntactic structures, such as:

a) 'Put the pen on the watch.'

b) 'Touch the watch with the pen.'

c) 'Touch the keys and then the pen.'

d) 'Touch the pen before touching the keys.'

e) 'Touch the pen but not the keys.'

f) 'Put the pen between the watch and the keys.'

g) 'You pick up the watch and give me the pen.'

h) 'Touch not only the pen but also the keys.', etc.

3. *Conceptual comprehension:* this can be tested using the same array f objects by asking questions such as these:

a) 'Point to the item used for recording the passage of time.'

(b) 'Touch the one used for writing.'

(c) 'Which of these items would you use for opening doors?'

Other similar conceptually-based questions are:

(d) 'What do you call the grey dust left after smoking a cigarette?

(e) 'What do you call the instrument we use for listening to the heart?'

(f) 'What do you call the bird that flies at night and hoots?'

(g) 'What is the hard outer case that protects animals like snails and tortoises?'

The most widely-used formal test of language comprehension is the Token Test, in which the subject has to follow commands of increasing syntactic complexity. The Peabody Picture Vocabulary Test is a picture–word matching test of single-word comprehension (see Appendix).

Repetition

Repetition should be tested with a series of words and sentences of increasing complexity. It is best to start with short single words, and then to progress to polysyllabic words and finally sentences. The sentences should include ones that are rich in small grammatical function-words, which are particularly difficult for aphasic patients. Patients can then be graded on their ability to repeat accurately. Phases such as 'no ifs, ands, or buts' are usually more difficult than sentences like 'The orchestra played and the audience applauded.'

Aphasics who cannot repeat have lesions involving the peri-sylvian language structures. Disproportionately severe breakdown of repetition is found in conduction aphasia. Lesions outside the primary language zone and progressive degenerative disorders spare repetition, producing what are termed transcortical aphasia syndromes (see p. 58).

Reading

Both reading aloud and reading comprehension are important, but must be carefully distinguished. Failure to comprehend is usually accompanied by incorrect reading aloud. On the other hand, there are many patients who cannot read aloud correctly, but have good understanding. If the patient successfully reads words and sentences, the capacity to read and understand a short paragraph should be tested. Simple reading comprehension can be tested by writing down a command such as 'Close your eyes' or 'Place your hands on top of your head if you're aged over sixty.' More complex comprehension can be assessed by asking the patient to read a paragraph from the newspaper and then asking questions about the content.

In most instances reading skills parallel spoken language abilities. But occasionally alexia may occur with agraphia, but without other aphasic deficits. Even more rarely, alexia may exist without even agraphia; this is called 'pure alexia' or 'alexia without agraphia' (see p. 61).

Once a reading problem has been uncovered, the next step is to determine which aspects of the normal reading process have broken down. The various types of dyslexia have been described (see p. 66), and consist of:

1. pure alexia: letter-by-letter reading;

2. neglect dyslexia; and

3. central (linguistic) dyslexias: surface, deep, etc.

Letter-identification

Errors in single-letter reading and the strategy of laboriously naming each letter (letter-by-letter reading), sometimes aided by tracing the letter outline with the finger, typify pure alexia.

Types of reading errors

Errors confined to the initial part of the word occur in neglect

dyslexia (for example, FISH for DISH) secondary to righ
hemisphere damage. Reading a word as another conceptuall
related, but not sound-related word (ACT for PLAY, SISTER fo
UNCLE, OCCASION for EVENT) is seen only in deep dyslexi
(see p. 64), in which visual errors are also common (SHOCK fo
STOCK, CROWD for CROWN, etc.).

Regular vs exception word reading

Selective difficulty reading words which do not obey the norma
sound-to-print rules of English—so-called 'exception words'—wit
a tendency to produce regularization errors (PINT to rhyme wit
MINT) is the defining characteristic of surface dyslexia (see p. 63

Non-word reading

Patients with deep dyslexia, in which there is a breakdown in th
sound-based reading route, are unable to read plausible non-word
(NEG, GLEM, HINTH, DEAK, etc.). In deep dyslexia othe
deficits are present; but in phonological dyslexia the only majo
problem is with reading these nonsense words.

   To screen for dyslexic syndromes, the list given in Table 4.
below, which contains non-words, regular words, and exceptio
words of mixed frequency, is suggested:

Table 4.1   A word-list for screening dyslexic syndromes

Exception words		Regular words		Non-words
Pint	Soot	Shed	Board	Neg
Gauge	Steak	Nerve	Bridge	Glem
Sew	Suite	Wipe	Gaze	Gorth
Naïve	Aunt	Ranch	Flame	Mive
Thyme	Tomb	Swerve	Mug	Rint
Mauve	Height	Hoarse	Vale	Plat
Epitome	Dough	Sparse	Pleat	Hinth
Cellist	Sieve	Scribe	Ledge	Deak

Writing

Writing ability can be analysed in terms of the manual execution of writing, recall of individual letters and words, and sentence composition. Three major types of dysgraphia are recognized (see p. 65):

1. dyspraxic dysgraphia;

2. neglect or spatial dysgraphia: line and word-based neglect; and

3. central (linguistic) dysgraphias: surface (lexical), phonological, and deep.

The type of writing disorder can usually be determined by spontaneous writing, writing to dictation, and oral spelling.

Spontaneous writing

It is usually sufficient to screen for dysgraphia by asking patients to compose a few sentences about a subject of their choice. If they are unable to think of anything, suggest a recent journey or a description of their home. Defects in letter formation, spelling, and grammatical composition should be readily apparant. If errors occur, then analysis of the specific deficit is required.

Note: it is not adequate merely to sample a patient's signature. Many severely dygraphic patients maintain the ability to write their name, which can be thought of almost as an automatic reflex activity.

Writing to dictation

To analyse the type of linguistic deficit in writing it is useful to have list which contains words with regular sound-to-spelling corres-ondence and words with exceptional spelling. The list suggested bove for reading will also serve this purpose.

Oral spelling

If the disorder of writing appears to be motoric, in that individual letters are poorly formed, reversed, or illegible, then it is useful to check oral spelling, which is normal in dyspraxic and neglect agraphias.

Calculation

Difficulty in writing, reading, and comprehending numbers, termed **acalculia**, should be distinguished from **anarithmetria**, in which basic numerical skills are preserved, but the patient is unable to perform arithmetical computations. The former most often occurs in association with aphasia; but the two may dissociate. The latter is common in dementia.

Assessment of the aphasic components of acalculia (number reading and writing) should be assessed first, by asking the patient to do the following:

(a) Write a series of simple (7, 2, 9, etc.) and complex (27, 93, 107, 1226, etc.) numbers to dictation.

(b) Read numbers aloud.

(c) Copy numbers.

(d) Point to numbers on command.

(e) Calculation skills should then be tested by asking the patient to perform oral arithmetic calculations which sample the four basic operations, i.e. addition, subtraction, division, and multiplication.

(f) Written calculations should then be examined.

(g) Finally, an examination should be made of arithmetical reasoning, such as 'If it takes two men three days to do a job, how long would it take four men to do the same job?'

Apraxia

Tests of apraxia can be divided according to the region of the body tested (buccofacial, limb) and the mode of examination (command, imitative). The use of real objects can also be assessed. Patients may be selectively impaired for movements of certain regions. Virtually all are impaired on command; but performance often improves when imitating the examiner A common error is the use of 'body-part-as-object', so that, for instance, when miming the use of a toothbrush, the forefinger substitutes as a brush, or when showing how to use a pair of scissors, the patient uses the index and middle fingers. A schedule for examining for buccofacial and limb gestures is shown on p. 151).

RIGHT-HEMISPHERE FUNCTIONS

Neglect phenomena

Personal
- Denial of existence of one side
- Denial of hemiplegia (anosagnosia)
- Unconcern about deficit (anosodiaphoria)

Sensory
- Visual, auditory, and tactile neglect
- Sensory extinction to simultaneous bilateral stimulation

Hemispatial neglect
- Freehand copying of symmetrical representational drawings (for example, a clock-face, a double-headed daisy, etc.)
- Visual search tests (for example, star cancellation)
- Line bisection

Neglect dyslexia and dysgraphia

- Line/page and word-based tests of reading and writing

Denial of hemiplegia (anosagnosia) and related conditions

Many patients with acute left hemiplegia do not realize that they are paralysed, and some frankly deny their deficit even when specifically challenged. This type of deficit is overlooked because examiners take it for granted that hemiplegic patients are aware that they are paralysed down one side. To detect these disorders, it is necessary to question all stroke patients about their deficits and to compare their subjective assessments with objective findings. The following hierarchy of denial phenomena can be applied:

1. denial of the existence one side, sometimes accompanied by somatic delusions, such as of the possession of three arms;

2. denial of hemiplegia, but not of the existence of the affected part (anosagnosia); and

3. realization of hemiplegia, but with an underplaying of its severity and the resultant disability (anosodiaphoria).

Manifestations of personal (bodily) neglect

Personal neglect may be apparent because a patient fails to groom one side of their head or shave one half of their face. Occasionally they have difficulty in dressing one side, or bump into objects on one side—usually the left. Head and eye deviation away from the neglected side (towards the lesion) implies damage to the frontal eye fields, and is a poor prognostic sign.

Sensory neglect

Patients with severe neglect may consistently ignore sensory inputs from the side contralateral to the side of their brain lesion. This usually occurs with right-sided lesions, so that the stimuli to the left are ignored. The following modalities should be tested.

Visual: The patient may ignore all visual stimuli to the contralateral side; if severe, this may be impossible to distinguish from hemianopia.

Auditory: The patient appears not to hear sounds to one side, and ignores visitors seated on that side of the bed.

Tactile: The patient ignores all sensory inputs from the affected side.

Sensory extinction to bilateral simultaneous stimulation

The patient responds when stimuli (visual, auditory, or tactile) are presented to one side, but when simultaneously stimulated from both sides consistently ignores the neglected side.

Extrapersonal (hemispatial) neglect

Neglect of one half of space is fairly common after damage to either hemisphere; but persistent severe hemispatial neglect is seen only after right-sided damage. The following tests can be used to detect neglect phenomena.

1. *Freehand copying of representational drawings* Items such as a clock-face, a flower-head, or a house are conventionally used, because they are two-dimensional and symmetrical. Another recently devised drawing, a two-headed daisy in a plant pot, has proved to be very useful in screening patients for unilateral neglect. Samples are shown below. It can be seen that patients with neglect omit or fail to complete one side (see Fig. 4.4). On the clock-face drawing, they either enter all the numbers on the right, or put in only the first six and omit the remainder (see Fig. 4.5).

If asked to copy an array of items (for example, a house, a tree, and a man) they complete only one half of each item (see Fig. 4.6). This phenomenon, referred to as **object-centred neglect**, demon-

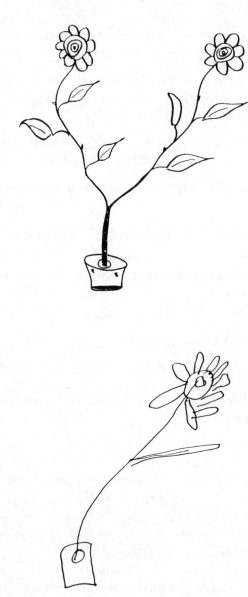

Fig. 4.4 Unilateral visual neglect: a right hemisphere stroke patient's attempt at copying the double-headed daisy, showing classic neglect of the left side (provided by Dr Peter Halligan).

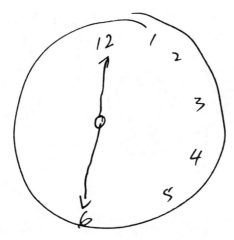

Fig. 4.5 The clock-face drawing of a patient with unilateral left-sided neglect following an acute right hemisphere stroke (provided by Dr Peter Halligan).

strates that the deficit is not a general neglect of the left half of space, but rather a specific defect in reconstructing the internal representation of individual objects.

2. *Visual search tasks*   Tests which require the subject to search a visual array for target shapes or letters are probably the most sensitive for detecting mild visual neglect. A recently devised version uses a mixture of words, letters, and stars of various sizes scattered randomly across a sheet of A4 paper. The subject is asked to cross out all the *small stars* (see Fig. 4.11, p. 153). An alternative version uses short lines at various angles scattered across a page. The subject is asked to cross out each of the lines.

3. *Line bisection*   Another traditional test of hemispatial neglect is to get the patient to mark the half-way point of lines of varying length, as shown on p. 152. Patients with neglect consistently bisect the lines to the right of the mid-point. The degree of displacement is directly proportional to the length of the line used, so that the phenomenon is easier to detect using longer lines.

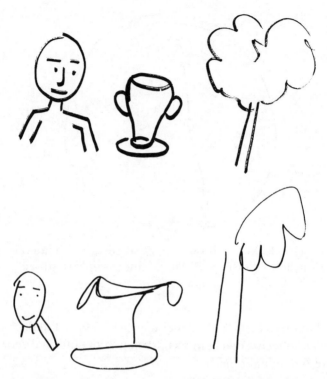

Fig. 4.6 Object-centred neglect: an example of a neglect patient's copy of three items in a single array (provided by Dr Peter Halligan).

Neglect dyslexia and neglect dysgraphia

These conditions are almost invariably associated with right-sided brain damage. Neglect dyslexia may affect lines of text or individual words. In the former, the patient omits the initial (left) part of each line, so that he or she reads only part of the text, rendering it nonsense. In the written equivalent, the patient writes on the right half of the page, and often leaves a progressively widening margin.

In word-based dyslexia, errors occur on reading the initial letters of words, which may be omissions (ISLAND to LAND) or substitutions (GRANT for PLANT). Word-based neglect dysgraphia causes the same type of errors, but in writing.

These syndromes are usually noted during language testing. But patients with other phenomena of neglect should be asked specifically to read a section of text from any book or magazine with wide columns. The word-list previously suggested to check reading and writing should also detect word-based neglect dyslexia and dysgraphia.

Dressing apraxia

This is best detected by questioning family members or nursing staff. It may be observed on the ward. If there is any suggestion of dressing difficulty, a good test is to observe the patient putting on a shirt/blouse which has been turned inside out.

Constructional ability

Drawing

- copying 3-D shapes (for example, a cube) and complex 2-D figures (for example, interlocking pentagons); and
- the Rey–Osterrieth Complex Figure Test (see p. 211).

Disorders of constructional ability are best detected by getting the patient to copy 3-D drawings, such as a cube, or a complex 2-D shape, such as the interlocking pentagons which form part of the Mini-Mental State Examination (see p. 186); even patients with quite severe impairment of constructional skills may be able to copy more simple shapes, such as a Greek cross (see Fig. 4.7). For a more stringent and quantitative test the Rey–Osterrieth Complex Figure Test is recommended, since the patient's copy can be scored using standard criteria (see Fig. 4.8). Delayed recall of the figure, usually after 30 to 40 minutes, can also be used as a measure of non-verbal memory.

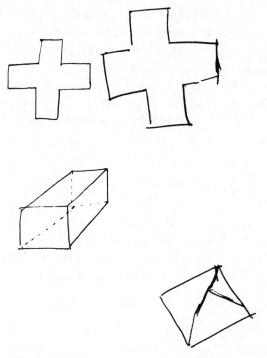

Fig. 4.7 The copy of a Greek cross and a cube by a patient with a right-sided lesion, showing preservation of simple drawing but an inability to copy the 3-D cube.

Complex visuo-perceptual abilities and the agnosias

Object recognition
- Description of visually presented objects

- Matching objects in arrays

- Copying of drawings of objects

- Object matching

- Verbal knowledge of objects

Tactile naming

Formal test: The Visual Object and Space Battery (see Appendix)

Prosopagnosia

Face description

Face recognition and naming

Face matching

Verbal knowledge of misnamed persons

Identification from voice, gait, etc.

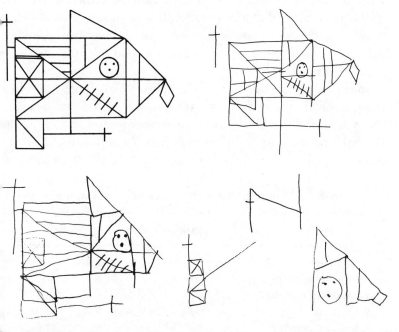

Fig. 4.8 The Rey–Osterrieth Complex Figure (upper left) and the copies of three patients with mild (upper right), moderate (lower left), and severe (lower left) impairment of constructional abilities.

Deficits in object and face recognition are difficult to assess at the bedside without special test materials; but if there are clues that some form of agnosia may be present the following relatively simple tasks can be employed.

Visual object agnosia

If the patient is unable to recognize simple objects or pictures despite good visual acuity and intact language abilities, a form of visual agnosia should be suspected.

In *apperceptual visual agnosia*, there is a breakdown at the stage of perceptual analysis, so that the patient is unable to describe the visually presented item and to match it with identical items. Patients' copies of drawings will be slow and fragmented, and identification of real objects is better than of photographs or of line-drawings. However, knowledge of the unidentified objects is preserved when tested verbally, and they can identify objects by touch (see p. 81).

In *associative visual agnosia* the perceptual stages of object recognition are preserved, but patients are unable to make sense of the visual information; object description and matching are normal, and they can copy line drawings. In most cases, the deficit represents a loss of semantic knowledge (see p. 16). This causes an

Table 4.2 Differentiating the forms of visual agnosia

	Apperceptive	Associative
Objective feature description	±	−
Visual identification	+	+
Copying line drawings	+	−
Object matching	+	−
Object knowledge	−	±
Tactile naming	−	±

+ affected; − spared; ± variable (usually affected).

1ability to name or identify items presented by any sensory 1odality, and a loss of verbal knowledge about the same items when sked probing questions.

Object feature description denotes the ability to describe the shape, utline, surface features, and colour of the presented object or icture.

Visual identification means the ability to recognize accurately the ttributes of the visually presented stimulus even if unable to roduce the name (for example, 'It's one of these things used by octors to listen to your heart.').

Copy line drawings is tested by asking the patient to copy drawings f representational items such as a flower, a bicycle, a house, etc.

Object matching describes the ability to match identical objects or ictures of objects. To test this it is necessary to use an array of items r pictures, two of which are identical. The patient is asked to point) the two items which are the same.

Object knowledge means the ability to generate accurate verbal escriptions when given the name of objects which the patient annot identify visually.

Tactile naming is tested by getting the patient to name objects by alpation with the eyes closed.

rosopagnosia

atients with severe deficits in visual analysis causing apperceptive gnosia are invariably impaired at recognizing faces. The syn-rome of prosopagnosia is a specific form of associative agnosia in which visual perception of faces, and hence the ability to describe nd match faces, is preserved, but there is a disorder of face ecognition and identification. In suspected cases the following unctions should be assessed.

. Face description—the ability to analyse and describe constituent facial features and expressions is preserved.

. Face recognition and naming is severely defective.

3. Face matching—the ability to match together identical faces o portrait photographs should also be preserved.

4. Knowledge of misnamed persons—in classic prosopagnosi. there is retention of knowledge about the famous people, friends and relatives, despite the inability to name them from photo graphs. A loss of knowledge about family and famous personal ities implies a disorder of semantic memory.

5. Identification from voice, gait, and dress is preserved.

Checklist for testing cognitive function

Global (non-localized) functions

1. **Alertness and general observations**

2. **Orientation**

Time	Time of day	—
	Day	—
	Date	—
	Month	—
	Year	—
Place	Building	—
	Town	—
Person	Name	—
	Age	—
	Date of birth	—

3. **Attention/concentration**
 (a) Months of the year backwards   No. of errors   —
   If failed, try days of the week backwards
 (b) Digit span: Read numbers at one per second without cluster
        ing.
        Discontinue after two failures at any level.

Span = highest sequence passed on either trial.

Forwards	*Backwards*
5—8—2	3—9
6—9—4	6—2
6—4—3—9	3—7—2
7—2—8—6	5—6—9
4—2—7—3—1	9—2—6—4
7—5—8—3—6	1—7—5—3
6—1—9—4—7—3	8—4—6—1—9
3—9—2—4—8—7	9—3—7—4—6
5—9—1—7—4—2—8	2—8—1—3—9—7
4—1—7—9—3—8—6	1—4—9—3—7—4

Span =   Span =
(normal 6 ± 1)   (normal 5 ± 1)

. **Memory**

ι) Anterograde   Name and address,   Peter Marshall
                   e.g.   42 Market Street
                                         Chelmsford
                                         Essex

               Immediate recall   First trial: correct   __/7
                                   Second trial   __/7
                                   Third trial   __/7
emember to test delayed recall after 5 minutes.   __/7

ɔ) Retrograde
Public events, e.g.   Recent sporting events
                      Royal family news
                      General election
                      Yugoslavian civil war
                      Russian coup
                      Gulf War

Resignation of Margaret Thatcher
Falklands War, etc.
Name of PM__;   Leader of the Opposition__;   President of USA__

5. **Frontal executive function**
(a) Initiation: verbal fluency
(i)   Letters: tell the patient that he or she will be asked to generate as many words as possible beginning with a letter, but that proper nouns (people and places, etc.) and variations of the same word (pass, passing, passed, etc.) are not allowed.
(ii) Animals: in the same way ask the patient to generate the names of as many animals as possible in one minute. These can begin with any letter.

Record all responses.

	'F'	'A'	'S'	Animals
Total	—	—	—	—
No. correct	—	—	—	—
Perseverations	—	—	—	—

(c) Abstraction: proverb interpretation
  • 'Still waters run deep.'
  • 'One swallow doesn't make a summer.'

d) Similarities

In what way are the following the same?   Response

- 'An apple and a banana'   _____
- 'A coat and a dress'   _____
- 'A table and a chair'   _____
- 'A poem and a statue'   _____
- 'Praise and punishment'   _____

e) Alternating sequences

Ask the patient to copy the following sample, and then to continue with the same pattern.

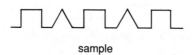

sample

f) Go–No-Go

Patient places hand on table and is asked to raise *one finger* in response to a single tap, but to hold still in response to two taps. The examiner taps the undersurface of the table.

Performance: _____

g) Motor sequencing

Luria three-step:

Demonstrate hand sequence (fist—edge—palm; see p. 122) five times, and than ask subject to repeat sequence.

_____

Alternating hand movements:

Demonstrate sequence five times (start position—one hand has fingers extended and the other has clenched fist, then positions alternate; see p. 122), and then get subject to copy.

_____

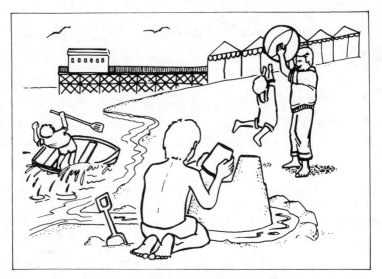

Fig. 4.9 The seaside scene from the Queen Square Screening Test for Cognitive Deficits: an example of a complex interactive scene for use in eliciting spontaneous language (reprinted by permission of Professor Elizabeth Warrington).

Localized cognitive functions

6. **Language**

(a) Spontaneous speech assessed on conversation and picture description:

- articulation
- fluency (phrase length)
- grammar
- word-finding
- paraphasic errors (phonemic or semantic)
- prosody

(b) Naming—10 items of varying familiarity   /1
e.g. pen, nib, watch, winder, buckle, stethoscope, etc.
Record errors

c) Comprehension

ingle words—point to objects in the room
e.g. bed, telephone, flowers, door, ceiling, etc.)

__/5

Grammar: using an array of 3 objects (e.g. pen, keys, watch)
  'Put the pen on the watch.'
  'Touch the watch with the pen.'
  'Touch the keys and then the watch.'
  'Touch the pen before touching the keys.'
  'Touch the pen but not the keys.'
  'Put the pen between the watch and the keys.'
  'You pick up the watch and give me the pen.'
  'Touch not only the pen but also the keys.'

__/8

Conceptual
  'Point to the item used for recording the passage of time.'
  'Touch the one used for writing.'
  'Which of these items would you use for opening doors?'
Other similar conceptually-based questions
  'What do you call the grey dust left after smoking a cigarette?'
  'What to you call the instrument we use for listening to the heart?'
  'What do you call the bird that flies at night and hoots?'

__/6

d) Repetition
Words: uncle, banana, tomorrow, artillery, orchestra, constitu-
onal

__/6

Phrases:
'The orchestra played and the audience applauded.'
'No ifs, ands, or buts.'   __/2

e) Reading aloud and comprehension
When the two boys set off to sail their dinghy to the nearby island
ie weather had been fine, but soon black clouds appeared in the

sky and a fierce wind began to blow. They turned around, and after almost capsizing, managed to get back to the shore, much to the relief of their waiting parents.'

If defective, or dyslexia suspected on other grounds:
Test single-letter identificaiton.
Administer word-lists, noting types of errors (visual, semantic phonemic).

Exception words		*Regular words*		*Non-words*
Pint	Soot	Shed	Board	Neg
Gauge	Steak	Nerve	Bridge	Glem
Sew	Suite	Wipe	Gaze	Gorth
Naïve	Aunt	Ranch	Flame	Mive
Thyme	Tomb	Swerve	Mug	Rint
Mauve	Height	Hoarse	Vale	Plat
Epitome	Dough	Sparse	Pleat	Hinth
Cellist	Sieve	Scribe	Ledge	Deak

(f) Writing
• spontaneous writing of a novel sentence
• writing to dictation
If defective, check written and oral spelling of the list above.

7. **Calculation** (if left hemisphere lesion suspected, see p. 132 for details)
Number reading and writing to dictation (8, 2, 27, 95, 236, etc.)
Oral and written arithmetic abilities
(e.g. $5+4$, $13+9$, $17+28$, $11-7$, $23-7$, $41-13$)

8. **Praxis**
Ask the patient to perform the following ('Show me how you would . . .').

f defective by command, test by imitation.

Command   Imitation

Buccofacial
  Blow out a match
  Lick lips
  Cough
  Sip through a straw

Limb
a) Gestures:
  Wave goodbye
  Beckon 'come here'
  Salute, like a soldier
  Hitch a lift
b) Object Use:
  Comb hair
  Brush teeth
  Use scissors
  Hammer a nail

. Neglect phenomena
a) If hemiplegic, assess degree of awareness of deficit.
b) Sensory neglect:
Test by extinction to bilateral simultaneous stimulation:
    tactile modality;
    visual modality.
c) Extrapersonal neglect
 Clock-face: get the patient to put in the numbers and set the
hands at quarter to two.

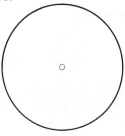

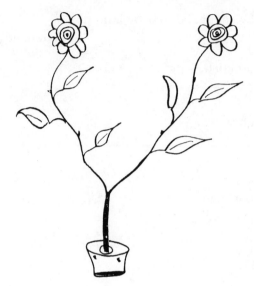

Fig. 4.10 Double-headed daisy in a pot.

- **Double-headed daisy:** ask the patient to copy the figure (Fig 4.10).
- **Visual search:** ask the patient to cross out all the *small* star (Fig. 4.11).
- **Line bisection:** ask the patient to mark the half-way point o each line with an *x*.

- **Neglect dyslexia and dysgraphia:** check for word- or line based neglect (see p. 138) if other features of extra-personal neglec are present.

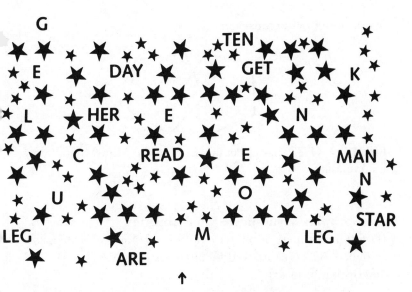

Fig. 4.11 Star Cancellation Test from the Behavioural Inattention Test (reprinted by permission of Thames Valley Test Company): the subject is asked to cross out all the small stars.

0. **Construction abilities** (ask the patient to copy the shapes below).

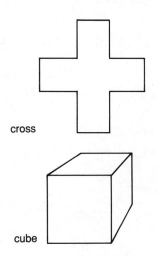

overlapping pentagons

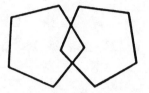

Fig. 4.12 Overlapping Pentagons from the Mini-Mental State Examination.

11. **Complex visuo-perceptual abilities**

If right hemisphere or bilateral posterior lesions suspected, assess fo evidence of perceptual difficulties as follows (see p. 142, fo description of tasks).

Object recognition
- Description of visually presented objects
- Matching of objects in arrays
- Copying of drawings of objects
- Object matching
- Verbal knowledge of objects
- Tactile naming

Prosopagnosia: If a disorder of face recognition is suspecte check:
- face description;
- face recognition and naming;
- face matching;
- verbal knowledge of misnamed persons; and
- identification from voice, gait, etc.

This chapter comprises twelve case histories written in short note form which illustrate the method of assessment proposed in Chapter 4. I have not attempted a comprehensive coverage of all cognitive disorders, but have selected a number of recent cases with either important common conditions (such as Alzheimer's disease) or interesting neuropsychological syndromes (such as prosopagnosia). Each case history is followed by a description of the findings on cognitive assessment, a brief differential diagnosis, and a summary of the principal conclusions, indicating whether the services of a neuropsychologist are required or not.

In most instances the results of both CT and functional brain scanning (SPECT) are also included. The latter technique, Single Photon Emission Computed Tomography, uses a radioisotope which crosses the blood–brain barrier and is taken up by brain cells. Photon emission reflects cerebral blood flow, and hence local metabolic rates. SPECT scanning is now widely available, whereas Positron Emission Tomography (PET), although a more sophisticated and sensitive functional imaging technique, is available in only a very few centres in the United Kingdom.

CASE 1 R.P.: 60-year-old farmer's wife

Diagnosis: EARLY ALZHEIMER'S DISEASE

History from patient: Aware of failing memory, which she has covered up by increasing use of memos and diary, etc. No features of depression (i.e. good energy level and enjoyment of life, no sleep disturbances, etc.).

History from family: One-year progressive decline in memory: especially evident for new information, with tendency to repetition. No obvious retrograde memory impairment. Preserved language and practical skills, but problems managing household accounts. No change in personality or behaviour.

Past medical history: Nil.

Physical signs: None.

Cognitive assessment

1. **General observations:** Normal appropriate behaviour, no mood disturbance.

2. **Orientation:** Normal, except date and day of week.

3. **Attention:** Normal
   Months of year backwards: Fast and accurate.
   Digit span forwards: 7
   Digit span backwards: 5

4. **Frontal executive functions:** Borderline.
   Verbal fluency: Mild reduction; F, A, S: 12 words per letter animals 10.
   Abstraction: Good interpretation of proverbs and similarities.

5. **Memory:** Impaired.
   Anterograde: Name and address registration: Normal; 7/7 first trial
   Recall: Poor; only 2 elements recalled after 5 minutes.
   Incidental recall of earlier conversation, etc.: Poor.
   Retrograde: Poor recall of recent news events.

6. **Language:** Borderline impairment in semantic component.
   Spontaneous speech: Fluent, normal articulation and syntax, no paraphasias.
   Comprehension: Normal even for complex commands.
   Naming: 7/10, three circumlocutions for parts of object (winder, nib, buckle).
   Repetition: Normal.
   Reading: Normal reading aloud and comprehension.
   Writing: Normal on spontaneous sentence.

7. **Calculation:** Normal.

8. **Praxis:** No deficit.

9. **Right hemisphere functions:** Normal, except Complex Figure Test.
   Neglect phenomena: Not present.

Visuo-constructive: Good copy of 3-D shape and overlapping pentagons, but impaired copying of Rey figure.

Visuo-perceptual: No deficits in object or face recognition.

Mental test scores

MMSE: 25/30. Above cut-off for 'dementia', lost points for recall of three items and two of the orientation questions.

Investigations

CT scan: Normal.

SPECT: reduced perfusion in bilateral temporo-parietal areas.

Differential diagnosis:

- Early Alzheimer's disease (see p. 37)

- Amnesic syndrome (see p. 12)

- Depressive pseudodementia (see p. 43)

Conclusions: This patient presented with features typical of early Alzheimer's disease, notably a fairly pure amnesic syndrome affecting episodic memory. The remainder of her cognitive function is generally well preserved, but other clues to the diagnosis are the reduced verbal fluency, the mild anomia, and the poor copy of a complex figure. Because of the importance of excluding a depressive pseudodementia a psychiatric opinion should be sought if there is any hint of affective symptoms. Similarly, a formal neuropsychological assessment is important to confirm the diagnosis.

Note:

- Insight often preserved early in Alzheimer's disease.

- Above 'cut-off' on MMSE.

CASE 2 A.B.: 75 year-old retired handyman

Diagnosis: MODERATE ALZHEIMER'S DISEASE

History from patient: Unaware of deficits, but when challenged admitted memory less good than he would expect.

History from family: Two to three years' insidious decline in memory; now unable to retain any new information. Very

repetitious. Grasp of recent events very poor, seems to 'live in th
past'. Recently having difficulty with household skills such a
cooking, and with hobbies, particularly gardening. Unable to g
shopping alone because of difficulty handling money. Speec
rather empty, with word-finding difficulty. Preserved social skil
and personality. No disturbance of mood. Initially some insight
but now fairly unaware of deficits.

Past medical history: Nil.

Physical signs: Normal.

Cognitive assessment

1. **General observations:** Good rapport, appropriate behav
   iour, well turned out, cheerful.

2. **Orientation:** Very poor: failed all five time orientatio
   questions; unaware of date, day, hospital'
   name, town, and county.

3. **Attention:** Mildly impaired.
   Months of the year backwards: Accurate but slow.
   Digit span forwards: 4
   Digit span backwards: 3

4. **Frontal executive functions:** Impaired.
   Verbal fluency: Very poor: F, A, S: 6 words per letter; animal
   5, with many perseverative responses.
   Abstraction: Poor proverb interpretation and similarities.

5. **Memory:** Severely impaired.
   Anterograde: Name and address registration: required three trials t
   recall all 7 elements.
   Recall: Nil recall after 10 minutes.
   Incidental recall of earlier conversation, etc.: very poor.
   Retrograde: Very poor grasp of past recent and news events
   muddled over own autobiographical details.

6. **Language:** Impaired semantic components and writing
   Spontaneous speech: Fluent and well articulated, with norma
   syntax; but empty, with word-finding diffi
   culty and circumlocutions.

Comprehension: Normal.

Naming: Reduced: 5/10, with circumlocutions for less common items (nib, strap, winder, buckle, stethoscope).

Repetition: Normal for words and sentences.

Reading: Normal for text and single words.

Writing: Impaired; poor spelling and sentence composition.

7. **Calculation:** unable to perform even simple mental arithmetic tasks.

8. **Praxis:** Normal.

9. **Right-hemisphere functions:** Impaired.

Neglect phenomena: Not present.

Visuo-constructive: Very poor of 3-D cube and overlapping pentagons.

Visuo-perceptual: No obvious deficit in object or face recognition.

Mental test scores

MMSE: 18/30. Well below 'cut-off'; failed most of orientation items, recall of three items, and copy of pentagons.

Investigations

CT scan: Mild generalized cortical atrophy, with ventricular enlargement.

SPECT: Marked bi-parietal hypoperfusion.

Differential diagnosis:

• Alzheimer's disease

• Other causes of dementia (see p. 34)

Conclusions: The cognitive examination revealed very obvious impairment of memory, language, abstract thinking, and constructional abilities typical of moderately advanced dementia of Alzheimer's type. In this instance, formal neuropsychological assessment is unnecessary.

Note:

• Despite severity of cognitive deficits, well-preserved social behaviour and personality.

CASE 3 D.A.: 67-year-old retired shop assistant

Diagnosis: DEPRESSIVE PSEUDODEMENTIA

History from patient: Aware of poor memory and concentration; denied any symptoms of 'depression', but admitted to poor sleep with early-morning waking, low energy, and a lack of interest in the home and family.

History from family: Well until 6 months before, then rapid decline in memory as well as a change in personality, with apathy and disinterest. Poor appetite and sleep pattern. Very complaining and irritable. No overt depression.

Past medical history: 'Nervous breakdown' 15 years previously required hospital admission.

Physical signs. None.

Cognitive assessment

1. **General observations:** Unconcerned and rather fractious, poor rapport, very distractible.

2. **Orientation:** Poor on all time items.

3. **Attention:** impaired, especially digits backwards.
   Months of year backwards: Slow; lost track several times.
   Digit span forwards: 5
   Digit span backwards: 2.

4. **Frontal executive functions:** Impaired.
   Verbal fluency: Reduced; F, A, S: 10 words per letter; animals 10.
   Abstraction: Attempt to test interpretation of proverbs and similarities evoked 'don't knows'

5. **Memory:** Impaired.
   Anterograde: Name and address registration: very poor, 2/7 first trial and 4/7 after third trial.
   > *Recall:* Poor; only 3 elements recalled after 5 minutes.
   Incidental recall of earlier conversation: Better than on formal testing.
   Retrograde: Poor recall of recent new events; when probed replied 'don't know' to most questions.

6. Language: Normal, except reduced output.

Spontaneous speech: Fluent; normal articulation and syntax; no paraphasic errors.

Comprehension: Normal.

Naming: 9/10, one circumlocution.

Repetition: Normal.

Reading: Normal.

Writing: Normal.

7. Calculation: Able to do simple arithmetic $(2+7)$, but not division or multiplication.

8. Praxis: No deficit.

9. Right hemisphere functions: Normal.

Neglect phenomena: Not present.

Visuo-constructive: Good copy of 3-D shape and overlapping pentagons.

Visuo-perceptual: No deficits in object or face recognition.

Mental test scores

MMSE: 22/30: lost points on orientation and recall.

Investigations

CT scan: Normal.

SPECT: Normal.

Differential diagnosis:

- Depressive pseudodementia (see p. 43)

- Dementia, especially subcortical type (see p. 35)

Conclusions: Clues to diagnosis in this case are the relatively acute onset; biological features of depression (sleep and appetite); the loss of interest in life; and the past psychiatric history. Many cognitive features are, however, indistinguishable from those of organic syndromes such as Alzheimer's. Subsequently the patient responded well to treatment with antidepressants. Formal neuro-psychological and psychiatric assessment are clearly essential in this case.

Note:

- Below cut-off on MMSE for 'dementia'.

- Impaired attention and registration.

- Memory worse on formal testing than informal observation suggest.

- Frequent 'don't know' responses.

CASE 4 F.M.: 64-year-old self-employed builder

Diagnosis: DEMENTIA OF FRONTAL TYPE

History from patient: Unaware of any problems, and denied symptoms even when directly confronted.

History from family: Six to twelve months' progressive personality change, with lack of motivation, poor judgement, erratic mood swings, lack of empathy over disabled son, and a tendency to crack inappropriate and puerile jokes. Increasing marital disharmony had led to a referral for counselling, since simple 'bedside' mental testing by GP failed to reveal any deficits.

Past medical history: Nil; no excess alcohol intake.

Physical signs: Positive frontal release signs (pout, palmomental, and grasp) only. Sense of smell preserved, discs normal.

Cognitive assessment

1. **General observations:** Jocular and unconcerned; rather dishevelled appearance, but attended well to examination.
2. **Orientation:** Normal.
3. **Attention:** Impaired digits backwards.
   Months of year backwards: Fast and accurate.
   Digit span forwards: 6
   Digit span backwards: 3
4. **Frontal executive functions:** Severely impaired.
   Verbal fluency: Very poor: F, A, S: average 8 per letter, including obscene words; animals 8, with numerous perseverations.
   Abstraction: Very poor interpretation of proverbs.
   Cognitive estimates test: produced numerous bizarre errors.

Response inhibition: Go–no-go—normal.

Alternating sequences—normal.

5. Memory: Borderline impairment.

Anterograde: Name and address registration: Normal: 7/7 recalled after 2nd trial.

Recall: Poor: 4/7 items recalled.

Incidental recall of interview, trip to hospital, etc.: Good.

Retrograde: No obvious deficit: good recall of recent and past news items.

6. Language: Normal.

Spontaneous speech: Fluent: well articulated, no paraphasias, normal syntax.

Comprehension: Normal, even for complex syntactic commands.

Naming: Normal: 10/10 correct.

Repetition: Normal for words and sentences.

Reading: Normal single-word and text reading.

Writing: Normal, although spontaneous sentence rather disinhibited: 'I love sex'.

7. Calculation: Normal.

8. Praxis: No limb or orobuccal apraxia.

9. Right hemisphere functions: Normal.

Neglect phenomena: Not present.

Visuo-constructive: Good copies of 3-D figures.

Visuo-perceptual: No deficit.

Mental test scores

MMSE 29/30.

Investigations

CT scan: Mild frontal atrophy, with enlargement of anterior part of lateral ventricle.

SPECT: Marked bi-frontal hypoperfusion.

Differential diagnosis: causes of frontal lobe dysfunction (see p. 23)

- Focal lobar atrophy (Pick's disease)

- Subfrontal meningioma

- After-effects of head injury
- Alcohol-related frontal dementia
- Huntington's disease
- Other basal ganglia degenerative disorders

Conclusions: This is a typical presentation of progressive frontal dysfunction, which in this case turned out to be due to focal lobar atrophy (Pick's disease). Formal neuropsychological assessment is mandatory, since the cognitive deficits on bedside testing are relatively slight (reduced backwards digit span, poor verbal fluency and abstraction).

Note:

- History from informant most important.

- Near-perfect performance on the MMSE.

CASE 5 B.Y.: 50-year-old accountant

Diagnosis: NEWLY PRESENTING HUNTINGTON'S DISEASE

History from patient: Unaware of any cognitive deficits; but admitted to excessive fidgetiness for several years.

History from family: Two years' insidious change in personality with lack of drive and motivation, originally diagnosed as depression. Problems coping at work, and disorganized personal finances. Decline in personal care and appearance. Twitchy facial and hand movements noted about the same time by family members.

Past medical history: Nil.

Family history: Father died in 40s of pneumonia, spent some time in psychiatric care with 'nervous depression'. Paternal grandmother had jerky movements. No explicit diagnosis of Huntington's disease.

Physical signs: Prominent choreiform movements of face, head and arms. Unsteady reeling gait, with typical finger-flicking. Unable to maintain tongue protrusion. Frontal release signs (pout, palmo-mentals) present.

Cognitive assessment

1. **General observations:** Flat affect; unconcerned. Dishevelled appearance.
2. **Orientation:** Normal.
3. **Attention:** Impaired.
   Months of year backwards: slow; lost track several times.
   Digit span forwards: 5
   Digit span backwards: 3
4. **Frontal executive functions:** Impaired.
   Verbal fluency: Poor: F, A, S: 10 words per letter; 10 animals, with perseverative responses.
   Abstraction: Poor performance on proverbs and similarities.
   Response inhibition: Normal on go–no go.
5. **Memory:** Mildly impaired
   Anterograde: Name and address registration: Poor; required 3 trials to register all items
   Recall: Reduced: 4/7 items after 5 minutes.
   Incidental recall of earlier conversation: Poor.
   Retrograde: Grasp of recent political events very sketchy, and below expected level.
6. **Language:** Borderline naming, dysarthric.
   Spontaneous speech: Mildly dysarthric and hesitant, but preserved phonology and syntax; no paraphasic errors.
   Comprehension: Normal, even for complex commands.
   Naming: Borderline 8/10 (failed on nib and winder).
   Repetition: Normal.
   Reading: Normal.
   Writing: Normal.
7. **Calculation:** No deficit.
8. **Praxis:** No limb or orobuccal apraxia.
9. **Right hemisphere functions:** Mildly impaired.
   Neglect phenomena: Not present.
   Visuo-constructive: Poor copy of 3D figures and interlocking pentagons.
   Visuo-perceptual: No obvious deficit.

Mental test scores
  MMSE: 27/30.
Investigations
  CT scan: Normal.
  SPECT: Not performed.
Differential diagnosis:

- Huntington's disease

- Wilson's disease

- Cerebral vasculitis, especially S.L.E.

- Other very rare causes of chorea and dementia, such as acanthocytosis, etc.

Conclusions: Although the patient presented with chorea and is unaware of any cognitive deficits, bedside testing shows features suggestive of fronto-striatal dysfunction. Initially the family history was said to be negative, but further investigation revealed tell-tale features of Huntington's disease (i.e. a family history of psychiatric illness and involuntary movement disorder). Formal neuropsychological and clinical genetic referral is essential.

Note:

- Cognitive abnormalities relatively subtle—mild attentional deficit, problems with executive function, borderline memory performance, and poor visuo-spatial ability.

- MMSE again above 'cut-off' for dementia.

- CT scan may show caudate atrophy, but usually only in clinically obvious cases.

CASE 6 P.S.: 65-year-old retired garage proprietor

Diagnosis: AMNESIC STROKE: BILATERAL THALAMIC INFARCTION

History from patient: Vague recall of hospital admission, but no insight into persistent memory disorder or change in behaviour. Claims to be on active service in the navy and currently at home on shore leave.

History from family: Six months prior to assessment admitted to hospital in coma—found in bed by wife, unrousable. Rapidly regained consciousness, but severely confused and disorientated. Complex and persistent confabulatory state; believes that it is wartime and that he is on active service. Virtually no recall of past forty years. Unable to lay down new memories. Complete lack of motivation and drive; previously very active, now watches TV all day.

Past medical history: Hypertension and smoking. No prior cerebrovascular events. Very modest alcohol intake.

Physical signs: Disordered eye movements, with paralysis of voluntary vertical gaze.

Cognitive assessment

1. **General observations:** Apathetic and unconcerned. No insight, but fully attentive.

2. **Orientation:** Severe disorientation: gives year as 1945, fails all time items.

3. **Attention:** Normal.
   Months of year backwards: Fast and accurate.
   Digit span forwards: 7
   Digit span backwards: 5

4. **Frontal executive functions:** Mildly impaired.
   Verbal fluency: Reduced, with numerous perseverations: F, A, S: 10 words per letter; animals 12.
   Abstraction: Normal interpretation of proverbs and similarities.
   Response inhibition: Normal.

5. **Memory:** Severely defective.
   Anterograde: *Name and address registration:* Normal: 6/7 first trial.
   Recall: Nil after 5 minutes, even when prompted.
   Incidental recall of conversation: Very poor.
   Retrograde: Extensive deficit affecting recall of personal episodic and public events back to the 1940s.

6. Language: Normal.
   Spontaneous speech: Normal fluent speech, with preserved phonology and syntax; no paraphasias.
   Comprehension: Normal.
   Naming: Normal: 10/10.
   Repetition: Normal.
   Reading: Normal.
   Writing: Normal.
7. Calculation: Normal.
8. Praxis: No limb or orobuccal apraxia.
9. Right hemisphere functions: Normal.
   Neglect phenomena: Not present.
   Visuo-constructive: Normal copy of 3D and Rey complex figures.
   Visuo-perceptual: No deficit.

Mental test scores
   MMSE: 21/30: Lost points for orientation, and on recall of three items.

Investigations
   CT scan: Normal at presentation.
   MRI: Symmetrical bilateral thalamic infarcts involving dorso-medial nuclear group.
   SPECT: Not performed.

Differential diagnosis: Acute onset of amnesic syndrome (see p. 12), arising from:

- Strokes, either bilateral thalamic or medial temporal

- Wernicke–Korsakoff's syndrome (B_1 deficiency), usually associated with alcoholism.

- Anoxic hippocampal damage following cardiac arrest, etc.

- *Herpes simplex* virus encephalitis

- Closed head injury

Conclusions: The presentation with coma, evolving into an amnesic state with profound anterograde and retrograde memory deficit, is typical of bilateral thalamic infarction. CT scanning is often normal immediately post-stroke, but a subsequent MRI demonstrated the classic lesion. All the vital memory structures are supplied from the posterior cerebral artery. In a high proportion of normal subjects both medial thalamic areas receive supply from a single penetrating artery. Formal neuropsychological assessment is clearly desirable in this case.

Note:

- Preservation of short-term (working) memory.

- Evidence of frontal dysfunction due to secondary frontal deafferentation.

- Eye movement disorder typical of this syndrome.

CASE 7 P.B.: 72-year-old retired company executive

Diagnosis: PRIMARY PROGRESSIVE APHASIA: NON-FLUENT TYPE

History from patient: Five years' gradual loss of spoken language abilities, leading to difficulties in public speaking and communication with friends and family. Use of telephone impossible. Also problems with written composition.

History from family: Confirmed above history, and that non-linguistic abilities remain unaffected. Still able to handle money, play golf, drive, go shopping, and perform DIY jobs. Recently comprehension also becoming impaired.

Past medical history: Nil.

Physical signs: None.

Cognitive assessment

1. **General observations:** Normal behaviour, well dressed, attentive to examination.
2. **Orientation:** Normal is tested by means of multiple choice.
3. **Attention:** Digit span impaired.
   Months of year backwards: Unable to perform.
   Digit span forwards: 3
   Digit span backwards: 2

4. **Frontal executive functions:** Impaired.

   Verbal fluency: Severely reduced: F, A, S: 3 words per letter animals 6.

   Abstraction: Difficulty assessing because of poor language skills

   Response inhibition: Alternating sequences normal.

5. **Memory:** Unable to assess formally because of aphasia.

   Anterograde: Name and address registration: Untestable.

   Recall: Untestable.

   Incidental recall of conversation, etc.: Appears good.

   Retrograde: Good grasp of current events if tested by multiple choice.

6. **Language:** Severely impaired phonological and syntactic components.

   Spontaneous speech: Non-fluent, hesitant, and slow, with poor articulation and simplified syntax; numerous phonemic paraphasic errors.

   Comprehension: Good at single-word and simple command level but poor for complex syntax.

   Naming: Poor: 2/10 common items; some benefit from phonemic cues.

   Repetition: Poor for sentences, but able to repeat simple words.

   Reading: Mirrors spoken language; single-word reading showed surface dyslexia pattern (i.e. impaired reading of irregularly spelt words, such as PINT, ISLAND, MAUVE, with regularization errors).

   Writing: Letters well-formed, some spelling errors, simplified grammar.

7. **Calculation:** Able to perform simple oral and written calculations.

8. **Praxis:** Normal orobuccal and limb praxis.

9. **Right hemisphere functions:** Normal.

   Neglect phenomena: Not present.

   Visuo-constructive: Normal copy of even complex figures (e.g. Rey figure).

   Visuo-perceptual: No deficits.

Mental test scores

   MMSE: 21/30, but if tested by multiple-choice recognition 28/30.

Investigations

   CT scan: Mild left perisylvian atrophy.

   SPECT: Marked left fronto-temporal hypoperfusion.

Differential diagnosis:

- Primary progressive aphasia (see p. 40)

- Tumours and other space occupying lesions

Conclusions: The presentation with a progressive loss of language output and relatively good comprehension is typical of this form of focal lobar atrophy (Pick's disease). The preservation of practical everyday abilities and of right hemisphere function separates this from a dementia. The nature of the language deficit (i.e. impaired phonology and syntax) is distinct from that found in Alzheimer's disease, where lexico-semantic problems predominate. Formal neuropsychological evaluation required to confirm normal non-verbal and general intellectual abilities.

Note:

- Superficial assessment might just lead to the mistaken conclusion that memory is equally impaired, since verbal memory is impossible to test.

- Digit span reduced because of impaired phonological processing.

CASE 8 J.L.: 62-year-old mining-company owner

Diagnosis: TEMPORAL LOBE PICK'S DISEASE WITH FEATURES OF SEMANTIC MEMORY LOSS (SEMANTIC DEMENTIA)

History from patient: Twelve-month history of problems with 'memory', by which he meant difficulty retrieving names of people, places, and things.

History from family: Twelve months or so progressive word finding difficulty, with impaired comprehension, especially fo names of people, but also of things. For instance, unable to orde from menus because of difficulty understanding names of foods Day-to-day event memory good, and no decline in practica abilities. Also apparent problems in face recognition.

Past medical history: Nil.

Physical signs: No abnormality detected.

Cognitive assessment

1. **General observations:** Good rapport, appropriate behav iour, well turned out.

2. **Orientation:** Normal for time; unable to name hospital o town.

3. **Attention:** Normal.
   Months of year backwards: Fast and accurate.
   Digit span forwards: 6
   Digit span backwards: 5

4. **Frontal executive functions:** Impaired.
   Verbal fluency: Very poor: F, A, S: 8 per letter; animals 5; othe categories also very reduced, but no perseve rations.
   Abstraction: Poor proverb interpretation and similarities.

5. **Memory:** Mildy impaired.
   Anterograde: Name and address registration: required three trials to recall all 7 elements.
   Recall: 5/7 after 10 minutes.
   Incidental: Surprisingly good memory of earlier conversations, etc.
   Retrograde: Unable to produce names of public figures, bu recalled some events in detail.

6. **Language:** Impaired semantic component.
   Spontaneous speech: Fluent and well-articulated, with normal syntax; but empty, with word-finding diffi culty and circumlocutions.

Comprehension: Normal for complex syntactic commands; but conceptual comprehension poor.

Naming: Reduced: 5/10, with circumlocutions for less common items.

Repetition: Normal for words and complex sentences.

Reading: Unable to read irregularly spelt words, making regularization errors (i.e. surface dyslexic).

Writing: Spelling poor.

. Calculation: No problems performing mental arithmetic.

. Praxis; Normal.

. Right hemisphere functions: Impaired face recognition.

Neglect phenomena: Not present.

Visuo-constructive: Excellent copies of 3-D cube, pentagons, and complex figures.

Visuo-perceptual: Unable to identify faces of famous people, but description of facial features and face matching normal. Also impaired at recognizing names. For instance, could not name John Major, and did not recognize the name.

Mental test scores

MMSE: 28/30.

Investigations

CT scan: Temporal lobe atrophy.

SPECT: Marked asymmetric temporal hypoperfusion.

Differential diagnosis: Temporal lobe dysfunction secondary to:

- Progressive focal lobar atrophy (Pick's disease)

- Alzheimer's disease

- Post-traumatic temporal lobe damage

- *Herpes simplex* encephalitis

Conclusions: The impairment in naming, verbal fluency, word comprehension, and face recognition is secondary to a breakdown in semantic memory, which in this case was due to progressive focal atrophy of the temporal lobes (Pick's disease). This syndrome has been called semantic dementia. Semantic memory impairment also

occurs in moderate stages of Alzheimer's, when episodic memor
loss is marked and visuo-spatial deficits are apparent.

Note:
- Deficit in face recognition not due to prosopagnosia.

- Above 'cut-off' for dementia on MMSE, despite profoun
  semantic memory impairment.

- Surface dyslexia is a consistent finding in semantic dementia

CASE 9 A.C.: 60-year-old publican

Diagnosis: ACUTE FLUENT (WERNICKE'S) APHASIA

History from patient: Referred to casualty with acute onset c
'confusion'. No sensible history obtainable.

History from family: Awoke on day of admission 'talkin,
rubbish', that is to say strings of unconnected words, with frequen
non-words. Apparently unaware of problem. Comprehensio
impaired.

Past medical history: Hypertension and diabetes. Smoker unti
recently. No evidence of alcohol abuse.

Physical signs: Difficulty examining because of lack of co
operation and comprehension. Suggestion of right-field defec
when tested by menace. No hemiparesis or drift of outstretche
arms. No head or eye deviation.

Cognitive assessment
1. **General observations:** Alert, talking almost continuously
   difficult to get to attend to tasks.
2. **Orientation:** Untestable; replies with his own name.
3. **Attention:** Untestable
   Months of year backwards: Unable to perform.
   Digit span: Unable to perform.
4. **Frontal executive functions:** Untestable.
5. **Memory:** Unable to assess because of severe aphasia.
6. **Language:** Severely impaired.
   Spontaneous speech: Fluent well articulated strings of words, wit

numerous phonemic paraphasias and neologisms.

Comprehension: Obeys simple body commands (close eyes, open mouth); unable to point to objects on command or to follow quite simple syntactic commands.

Naming: 0/10, producing neologisms; no improvement with phonemic cues.

Repetition: Unable to get to perform.

Reading: Exactly parallels spoken language, and bears no obvious relationship to text.

Writing: Able to write own name, but not words to dictation.

. **Calculation:** Not attempted.

. **Praxis:** Follows mimed actions accurately.

. **Right hemisphere functions:** Normal.

Neglect phenomena: Not present.

Visuo-constructive: Copies simple shapes, but impaired copy of 3D geometrical shapes (cube).

Visuo-perceptual: No apparent deficit.

Mental test scores

MMSE: Not administered, in view of severe aphasia.

Investigations

CT scan: Initially normal, later confirmed infarct involving left superior temporal region.

SPECT: Not done.

Differential diagnosis: Causes of acute aphasia (see p. 46):

- Strokes: Infarction in middle cerebral artery territory or haemorrhage

- Abscess

- Encephalitis

- Space occupying lesions

- Head injury

Conclusions: The features are characteristic of an acute fluent aphasia of Wernicke's type secondary to an infarct involving the

superior temporal lobe (posterior branch, middle cerebral artery
The presence of a severe comprehensional deficit renders much
the cognitive assessment impossible. Formal neuropsychologic
referral is unnecessary at this stage.

Note:

- It may be difficult to distinguish acute fluent aphasia fro
  confusional states, and even mania; but the presence
  language errors on spontaneous speech and writing clinch
  the diagnosis.

- Wernicke's aphasia often occurs without physical signs.

CASE 10 F.B.: 40-year-old music teacher

Diagnosis: RIGHT PARIETAL TUMOUR

History from patient: Three months poor co-ordination
bumping into things to the left, and difficulty in playing the flut
No headaches or seizures.

History from family: As above; but family also concerne
about vagueness and poor concentration.

Past medical history: Nil.

Physical signs: No visual field defect, but neglect of left side
stimulus on bilateral stimulation. Also left tactile extinction
astereognosis, and graphasthesia.

Cognitive assessment

1. **General observations:** Rather slow and vague, but otherwis
   normal.
2. **Orientation:** Normal.
3. **Attention:** Impaired reverse digit span.
   Months of year backwards: Slow but accurate.
   Digit span forwards: 7
   Digit span backwards: 4
4. **Frontal executive functions:** Normal.
   Verbal fluency: Normal: F, A, S: 20 words per letter; animals 25
   Abstraction: Normal proverbs and similarities.
   Response inhibition: Not tested.

5. **Memory:** Normal.
   Anterograde: Name and address registration: Normal: 7/7 first trial.
   Recall: 7/7 after 10 minutes.
   Incidental recall: Normal.
   Retrograde: Accurate and detailed account of public events.
6. **Language:** All normal.
7. **Calculation:** Normal.
8. **Praxis:** No deficit.
9. **Right hemisphere function:** Severely impaired.
   Neglect phenomena: Present on drawing clock-face and two-headed daisy, star cancellation and line bisection.
   Visuo-constructive: Very disorganized copies of even simple 3-D figures (e.g. cube).
   Visuo-perceptual: No apparent deficit in object and face recognition.

Mental test scores
   MMSE: 28/30.

Investigations
   CT scan: Large intrinsic right parietal tumour.
   SPECT: Not done.

Differential diagnosis:
- Tumours (intrinsic or extrinsic)
- Abscess
- Other rarer space occupying lesions (e.g. tuberculoma, etc.)

Conclusions: This is a typical presentation of an intrinsic right posterior space occupying lesion. Formal neuropsychological assessment is not required.

Note:
- It is easy to miss the cognitive deficits if they are not specifically tested.
- Vagueness and slowing are often noted by observers, but there are virtually no specific accompanying signs except poor reverse digit span.

CASE 11 S.E.: 60-year-old retired railway-worker

Diagnosis: PROSOPAGNOSIA AND TOPOGRAHICAL MEMORY DEFICIT

History from patient: Since admission to hospital three years before with encephalitis, severe 'memory' problems, consisting of inability to recognize all but very familiar faces, and difficulty in navigating around even well-known places. Also severe loss of smell and taste.

History from family: Confirms above, and that his day-to-day memory (episodic) memory is very good. No problems with remote memory. Since his illness the patient is prone to uncontrolled emotional outbursts.

Past medical history: Nil.

Physical signs: Nil, except complete anosmia.

Cognitive assessment

1. **General observations:** Alert and attentive.
2. **Orientation:** Completely normal time and place.
3. **Attention:** Normal.
   Months of year backwards: Fast and accurate.
   Digit span forwards: 6
   Digit span backwards: 5
4. **Frontal executive functions:** Normal.
   Verbal fluency: Normal: F, A, S: 18 words per letter; animals 22; no perseverations.
   Abstraction: Good interpretation of proverbs.
5. **Memory:** Normal
   Anterograde: Name and address registration: 7/7 first trial.
   Recall: 6/7 after 10 minutes.
   Incidental: Good.
   Retrograde: Accurate and detailed recall of past personal and public events.
6. **Language:** Normal.
   Spontaneous speech: Fluent: well-articulated, with preserved phonology and syntax. No paraphasias.

Comprehension: Normal.

Naming: 10/10.

Repetition: Normal.

Reading: Normal.

Writing: Normal.

. **Calculation:** Normal.

. **Praxis:** Not tested.

. **Right hemisphere functions:** Severely impaired face recognition.

Neglect phenomena: Not present.

Visuo-constructive: Good copies of 3D shapes and complex geometrical figures.

Visuo-perceptual: Unable to name or identify face names, but normal on face feature description and choosing examples of the same face in arrays (matching tasks). Knowledge of famous people (from name) preserved (e.g. 'Who is John Major?'). Also unable to name or identify famous buildings. Naming and identification of objects normal.

Mental test scores

MMSE: 30/30.

Investigations

CT scan and MRI: Severe atrophy of right temporal lobe, involving hippocampus and temporal cortex, with enlarged right lateral ventricle. Left side normal.

SPECT: Not performed.

Differential diagnosis: Causes of prosopagnosia (see p. 86):

- *Herpes simplex* virus encephalitis

- Posterior cerebral artery territory stroke

- Penetrating head injury

- Carbon monoxide poisoning

Conclusions: This man's complaints of difficulty in face recogn
tion (prosopagnosia) and non-verbal memory suggest right ten
poral lobe dysfunction, which in this case is secondary t
asymmetrical destruction from *Herpes simplex* encephalitis. Bedsid
testing points to a true prosopagnosia rather than to a perceptiv
deficit or a loss of semantic memory underlying the face recognitio
deficit. Formal neuropsychological assessment is clearly importan
to clarify the deficits.

Note:

- Non-verbal memory is difficult to assess at the bedside.

- Normal constructional abilities, which depend on parietal lob
  function.

- Anosmia from olfactory bulb or entorhinal cortex damage.

CASE 12 J.R.: 75-year-old widow

Diagnosis: ACUTE CONFUSIONAL STATE (DELIRIUM)
URINARY INFECTION AND URAEMIA

History of patient: None available.

History from family: Two weeks' fluctuating confusion, wit
episodes of drowsiness. Disorientation in place, especially at nigh
with agitation and transient visual hallucinations. Poor memory fo
new information.

Past medical history: Rheumatoid arthritis, asthma, long-term
corticosteroid therapy.

Physical signs: Evidence of arthropathy and iatrogenic Cush
ing's syndrome. No focal neurological signs.

Cognitive assessment

1. **General observations:** Patient bemused, mildly drowsy, and
   very poorly attentive and distractible, occasionally picking a
   bedclothes.
2. **Orientation:** Poor: disorientated in time and place, but no
   person.

. **Attention:** Very impaired.

Months of year backwards: Unable to perform, loses sequence recurrently.

Digit span forwards: 3

Digit span backwards: 2

Frontal executive functions: Impaired.

Verbal fluency: Reduced: F, A, S: 5 words per letter, with intrusions and perseverations; animals 8.

Abstraction: Unable to interpret proverbs or perform similarities.

. **Memory:** Impaired.

Anterograde: Name and address registration: Very poor; unable to retain even after 3 trials.

Recall: Poor: 3/7 after 10 minutes.

Retrograde: Grasp of recent and past events reasonable if able to hold attention.

. **Language:** Essentially normal, except content.

Spontaneous speech: Fluent: well articulated, with good syntax, and no paraphasic errors; but rambling and inconsequential.

Comprehension: Normal, except for complex commands.

Naming: Normal: 9/10.

Repetition: Normal.

Reading: Normal.

Writing: Poorly formed and disorganized.

. **Calculation:** Unable to perform mental arithmetic, but number reading and writing normal.

Praxis: Normal.

Right hemisphere functions: Mild impairment.

Neglect phenomena: Absent.

Visuo-constructive: Poor copies of 3D shapes and overlapping pentagons.

Visuo-perceptual: No deficit apparent in face or object recognition.

Mental test scores

　MMSE: 18/30.

Investigations: Revealed urinary tract infection and mild degr
of renal failure.

　CT scan: Normal.

　SPECT: Not performed.

Differential diagnosis: Causes of delirium or acute confusion
state (see p. 31)

Conclusions: The history and cognitive features in this case a
characteristic of an acute confusional state (delirium), wi
impaired attentional processes resulting in poor memory proces
ing. Note also the poor visuo-spatial function. Formal neuropsych
logical assessment is not required.

Note:

- Impaired attention the major cognitive deficit.

Standardized mental test schedules: their uses and abuses

Introduction

A large number of mental test schedules have been used, which range in complexity from the ten-item Hodkinson Mental Test, which takes only moments to complete, to the much more complex Dementia Rating Scale (DRS), which takes 30 minutes or more to administer. For practical purposes however, they can be divided into two broad groups: (i) the brief schedules which can easily be used in the clinic, or at the bedside, and do not require any specialized equipment or training, and (ii) the more elaborate scales, which are used largely, at least at present, in research studies, and require the purchase of test materials and some training in their administration.

Because of the plethora of potential tests, I have chosen three of the most commonly used brief assessment schedules—the Mini-Mental State Examination (MMSE), the Information–Memory–Concentration Test (IMC), and the ten-item Hodkinson Mental Test, which is derived from the IMC. I have also chosen two longer tests which are now widely used in dementia research—the Mattis Dementia Rating Scale (DRS) and the CAMCOG.

These schedules all have limitations and are open to abuses; but this applies particularly to the shorter tests. They are undoubtedly useful for screening large populations, since they have good inter-rate reliability and fairly well-established normative data; but the results must be interpreted with caution when applied to individual patients. A number of general points deserve consideration before each test is described.

All the schedules sample a number of different areas of cognitive ability (for example, attention/concentration, memory, language, visuo-spatial abilities, etc.); hence failure can be due to various combinations of cognitive impairment. A low score may reflect appalling performance in one domain only, or slight impairment across all the domains evaluated. As a practical example, consider a score of 25 out of 30 on the MMSE. This could be due to a loss of all five points in the attention subset, or a loss of one or two points for each of orientation, attention, memory, and language. Both patterns produce the same total score, but the former is clearly much more significant. This illustrates how essential it is to consider the profile of performance on these tests, and not just the overall total score.

It should be emphasized that all the schedules were developed with a view to quantifying the cognitive failings in elderly subjects with dementia and/or delirium. They may, with certain provisos, be reliable measures in these situations; but this does not mean that they can be applied generally to patients with all types of cognitive impairment, both focal and general, acute and chronic. Of particular note is their insensitivity to circumscribed cognitive deficits. This is exemplified in patients with extensive right hemisphere lesions, who may have very major visuo-spatial and perceptual deficits, but score almost perfectly on any of the mental test schedules under consideration. They are also notoriously insensitive to frontal lobe disorders, and patients with disabling and profound deficits in 'executive' and social functions typically perform normally.

It should also be realized that the normative values and 'cut-off' levels generally applied in these tests veer towards specificity, rather than sensitivity, in dementia. A score below the cut-off of 24 on the MMSE (in the absence of features of delirium) is a fairly good marker of dementia. However, many patients with early Alzheimer's disease score above this cut-off, particularly if they are young and of superior background intellectual ability.

This brings up the important question of considering back ground demographic features which are likely to affect perform

nce. Age, education, and socio-economic status are the most
nportant variables. Ethnic group and first language should also be
onsidered. These factors are additive, so that the lower limit of
ormal for an elderly person with only a few years education is
adically different to that of a young, highly educated professional.
These points will be discussed further in relationship to the test
chedules under consideration.

Mini-Mental State Examination (MMSE)

nstructions: Record response to each question.

Domain tested	Score
Orientation	
Year, month, day, date, season	__/5
Country, county (district), town, hospital, ward (room)	__/5
Registration	
Examiner names three objects (e.g. orange, key, ball).	
Patient asked to repeat three names.	
Score one for each correct answer.	__/3

Then ask patient to repeat all three names three times.

Attention	
Subtract 7 from 100, then repeat from result, etc.	
Stop after 5: 100, 93, 86, 79, 72, 65 (do not correct if errors made).	
(Alternative if unable to perform serial subtraction: spell 'world' backwards: D L R O W.]	
Score the best performance on either task	__/5
Recall	
Ask for the names of the three objects learned earlier.	__/3
Language	
Name a pencil and a watch.	__/2
Repeat 'No ifs, ands, or buts'.	__/1

- Give a three-stage command. Score one for each stage (e.g. 'Take this piece of paper in your right hand, fold it in half, and place it on the chair next to you.').
- Ask patient to read and obey a written command on a piece paper stating: 'Close your eyes.'
- Ask patient to write a sentence. Score if it is sensible, and has a subject and a verb.

Copying

- Ask patient to copy intersecting pentagons.

Total score __/3

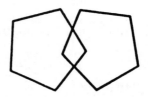

Fig. 6.1 Overlapping Pentagons from the Mini-Mental State Examination

The MMSE, designed by Folstein and colleagues from Baltimore, the most widely used and studied screening measure of cognitiv impairment. It has the advantages of brevity, ease of administra tion, and high inter-rater reliability. It can be easily incorporate into routine clinical practice, and provides a good rough-and-read screening test for dementia and delirium. It is also of practical valu in monitoring progression in these disorders. It is not usefu however, for the detection of focal cognitive deficits (amnesi aphasia, visuo-spatial disorders etc.), and is insensitive to front lobe disorders.

A score of less than 24 (i.e. a cut-off of 23/24) was initiall suggested for distinguishing between impaired and normal subjec (respectively) with a reasonably high degree of specificity an sensitivity. However, these values were derived from screenin elderly hospitalized patients with delirium or fairly advance

egrees of dementia, not outpatients with mild disease. Mild cases
ith early, but clinically definite, Alzheimer's disease score above
iis level. It has also been clearly established that the MMSE is very
ulnerable to the effects of age, education, and socio-economic
atus. The following age-related cut-offs have been proposed:

)s—29; 50s—28; 60s—28; 70s—28; 80s—26.

Further adjustments are required for educational level, especially
1 the older age-groups. For subjects aged over seventy who left
:hool before the age of fifteen (i.e. those with less than ten years of
lucation), a score of up to three less than the age-related score
iven above is acceptable as normal.

There are also difficulties with scoring the attentional subtest.
'he authors of the MMSE originally suggested that the spelling of
ie word WORLD backwards should be given to those unable to
erform serial subtraction. However, this instruction is rather loose,
nd leads to confusion. We have tended to administer serial sevens,
nd if *any* errors occur give subjects the task of spelling WORLD
ackwards. The score is then taken as the best performance on
ither of these two. Other authors have opted to give either the
:rial seven or the WORLD backward test to each subject.

The subtests most useful in detecting relatively early Alzheimer's
isease are the recall of the three items, followed by orientation and
rawing. The language tests are the least sensitive. In Huntington's
isease and other forms of subcortical dementia, the attentional
ibtests are those most vulnerable to disease. The MMSE is
isceptible to 'floor effects' in severely demented cases. That is to
iy, once patients reach a fairly advanced stage of disease they tend
) score very few points, and beyond this progression cannot be
ssessed.

Information–Memory–Concentration Test: American modification by Fuld

Instructions: One point for each correct answer unless otherwise indicated.

Domain tested   **Score**

Information
- Name
- Age
- Time (hour)
- Time of day
- Day of week
- Date
- Month
- Season
- Year
- Place: name
            street
            town
- Type of place (for example, home, hospital, etc.)   Total 1

Memory (NB: Administer name and address at this stage)
Personal
- Date of birth
- Place of birth
- School attended
- Occupation
- Mother's first name   Total
Non-personal
- Date of First World War 1914–1918 (half point if
  either date within 3 years)
- Date of Second World War 1939–1945 (half point if
  either date within 3 years)
- President (or Prime Minister)
- Past President (or past Prime Minister)   Total

Five-minute recall of name and address (score 0–5 points)
e.g. Mr John Brown
        42 West Street
        Gateshead   Total 5
Concentration (all scored 0—1—2)
● months of the year backwards
● Counting 1–20
● Counting 20–1   Total 6
                                            Maximum error score 33

The IMC, first published in 1968 as part of the Blessed Dementia Rating Scale, has been widely used and adapted since. The version shown is the American adaptation by Fuld, which has been well validated. The popularity of the IMC owes much to the fact that it remains virtually the only scale for which performance has been correlated with neuropathological parameters of severity in Alzheimer's disease, namely density of plaques and levels of choline acetyltransferase in post-mortem brains.

Its advantages, uses, and limitations are, in principle, the same as those of the MMSE, although the effects of age, education, and socio-economic status on it have not been as thoroughly evaluated. Because of the heavy weighting towards memory it is perhaps more sensitive to the early changes of Alzheimer's disease than the MMSE, although a number of studies have shown that performance on the two tests is closely correlated. Unlike other mental test schedules, the IMC is scored as the total number of errors, with a maximum of 33 in the Fuld version shown. More than 4 errors (i.e. a cut-off of 4/5) has been considered abnormal. But the cut-off should certainly be higher for the very elderly with low educational attainment, and should perhaps be even lower for young professionals.

Because of the emphasis on orientation and attentional tasks it is theoretically a good initial screening tool for acute confusional states (delirium), although this has not been well studied.

Hodkinson Mental Test

Instruction: Score one point for each question answered correctly.

Question	Score
• Age of patient	——
• Time (to nearest hour)	——
• Address given, for recall at end of test: 42 West Street	——
• Name of Hospital (*or* area of town if at home)	——
• Year	——
• Date of birth of patient	——
• Month	——
• Years of First World War	——
• Name of Monarch (President in USA)	——
• Count backwards from 20–1 (no errors allowed, but may correct self)	——
Total	/10

Derived from the Blessed Information–Concentration–Memory this test has been fairly widely used and validated for use with the elderly, but has not been studied to anything like the extent of the MMSE. The major, and arguably the only, point in its favour is its extreme brevity. An overall score of 6/10 or less is said to be abnormal in the elderly. Values for younger patients have not been established. Clearly not all questions are equivalent, and, as with other schedules, the profile of scores should be considered. It has no major advantages over the MMSE and IMC. If a brief screening schedule is required for general clinical use, I would favour one of these other tests.

Dementia Rating Scale (DRS)
(Published by NFER–Nelson.)

DRS Subtests	Score
Attention subtest	
Digit span (forwards and backward)	8
Two-step commands	2
One-step commands	4
Imitation of commands	4
Counting As	6
Counting randomly arranged As	5
Reading a word-list	4
Matching figures	4
	(37)
Initiation subtest	
Fluency for supermarket items	20
Fluency for clothing items	8
Verbal repetition (e.g. bee, key, gee)	2
Double alternating movements	3
Graphomotor (copy alternating figures)	4
	(37)
Construction subtest	
Copy geometrical designs	6
	(6)
Conceptualization subtest	
Similarities	8
Inductive reasoning	3
Detection of different item	3
Multiple-choice similarities	8
Identities and oddities	16
Create a sentence	1
	(39)
Memory subtest	
Recall a sentence (I)	4
Recall a self-generated sentence (II)	3

Orientation (e.g. date, place)	9
Verbal recognition	5
Figure recognition	4
	(25)

Total score 144

Originally designed by Mattis for use in a prospective study of dementia, the DRS assesses a fairly wide range of cognitive abilities, and contains a sufficient number of less demanding items that valid and reliable information can be obtained in more severely demented subjects. Its principal use is in research, particularly that involving longitudinal studies of demented patients or the comparison of patients with different pathologies.

It is easy to administer and score. The first four sections—attention, intiation, construction, and conceptualization—are graded in difficulty, and contain screening tests at the beginning. If these are passed, the remainder of the section need not be administered. The final memory section is given to all subjects. Approximately 20–40 minutes are required to administer it to demented patients, depending upon their level of impairment.

The DRS has been most widely used in patients with Alzheimer's disease. It is more sensitive to early disease than the brief scales discussed above, and shows less marked floor effects. It may also be helpful in distinguishing between different dementing illnesses. The memory section is most sensitive to Alzheimer's, whereas patients with Huntington's disease are most impaired on the initiation subtest. It should, in theory, be sensitive to the deficits seen on dementia of frontal type. Its usefulness in other forms of dementia remains to be seen.

Normal elderly subjects perform well on the DRS. The mean total score in a number of studies has ranged from 137 to 140. Our own experience, together with that of the San Diego Alzheimer's disease research group, suggests a cut-off of 131/132 for separating impaired from normal subjects. It is likely to be vulnerable to the same age, education, and socio-economic effects as the MMSE; but wide-scale community-based studies to establish more generally applicable normative values have not been performed.

It should also be noted that the DRS provides a broad test of the distributed cognitive functions (attention, memory, and abstraction/conceptualization), but includes virtually no assessment of localized functions, especially language.

Cambridge Cognitive Examination: CAMCOG
(Published by Cambridge University Press.)

CAMCOG subtests	Scores
Orientation	
Time—day, date, month, year, season	
Place—county, town, street, floor, place	10
Language	
Comprehension	
Naming of objects and pictures	
Expressive vocabulary	
Repetition	
Verbal fluency	
Reading comprehension	30
Memory	
Registration	
Recall—pictures, three items, name and address	
Recognition—pictures	
Remote memory	27
Attention	
Counting backwards and serial 7s	7
Praxis	
Copying and drawing	
Ideomotor gestures	
Writing—spontaneous and to dictation	12
Calculation	2
Abstract thinking—similarities	8

Perception
  Visual—faces and objects
  Tactile   1]
                                                       Total 10?

The Cambridge Cognitive Function Examination—CAMCOG—
forms part of a standardized psychiatric assessment schedule
CAMDEX, devised by Roth and colleagues and now published by
Cambridge University Press. CAMDEX was designed specifically
for use in elderly people with the diagnosis of dementia. It includes
a structured psychiatric interview with the patient, and a relative or
other informant interview; a brief physical examination; and a
neuropsychological test battery, CAMCOG.

CAMCOG assesses a wider range of cognitive functions, both
distributed (attention, memory, abstraction) and localized
(language, praxis, etc.) than any other standardized schedule. It
incorporates both the MMSE and IMC within the battery. The
average administration time is 20–40 minutes, depending on the
degree of impairment. There are 60 items, which yield eight
subscale scores. The maximum overall score is 107. A cut-off of
79/80 was found to discriminate between demented and normal
subjects, respectively, on the original validation studies with a high
degree of specificity and sensitivity. Further work has shown that, in
keeping with other mental test schedules, the normal range varies
considerably with age, and age-appropriate normative values are
now available.

CAMCOG is currently used extensively in community-based
studies of dementia, and is likely to become the best validated and
normed of the longer mental test batteries. The value of CAMCOG
in distinguishing between patients with various types of dementia
(cortical vs subcortical, etc.) has not been established.

In comparison with the DRS, CAMCOG is likely to be more
sensitive to mild degrees of dementia, and should be better at
detecting patients with predominant language or visuo-spatial
dysfunction; the DRS contains no language tests, and limited

assessment of drawing ability. A disadvantage of CAMCOG is the relative lack of very easy items, so that it is unlikely to be as valuable as the DRS for monitoring progress in patients with moderately severe dementia. Also it may not be sensitive to frontal lobe dysfunction; the attentional tests are extremely easy, and the abstraction subtest is limited.

Appendix: Neuropsychological tests

A large number of neuropsychological tests are commercially available. Many more, designed initially by psychologists for their own clinical and/or research purposes, have become fairly widely used, but are not published. In this section, I describe only a fraction of the tests potentially available. The ones I have chosen to describe are either (i) tests so commonly used by professional neuropsychologists (for example, the Wechsler Intelligence and Memory Scales) that clinicians interested in cognitive function should be aware of their make-up and scoring, if they are going to interpret neuropsychological reports (these tests are, on the whole, fairly time-consuming, and require training in administration, scoring, and interpretation); or (ii) tests that can be regularly used in the clinic or ward, that do not require special training, and that are relatively quick to administer and score (for example, digit span, story recall, Rey figure copy and recall, letter and category fluency tests, etc.). The tests are arranged in alphabetical order. Normative data are given as means with standard deviations (shown as $X \pm Y$). In the case of those tests which are professionally produced and copyrighted, I have given the name of the publishers. The address of the major test publishers are listed at the end of the Appendix.

The Autobiographical Memory Interview (AMI) (Thames Valley Test Company)

The AMI was designed by Kopelman, Wilson, and Baddeley to assess personal remote (retrograde) memory. There are two sections—the personal semantic schedule and the autobiographical incident schedule. In the first section, subjects are asked to recall specified *facts* from each of three epochs: childhood (for example, names of teachers and school), early adult life (for example, name of first employer, date and place of wedding), and recent life (for example holidays, journeys, and hospitalizations). Each of these is scored for accuracy. The second section assesses remote episodic memory. Subjects are asked to recall three specific *incidents* from each of the same life-periods. Scoring is in terms of the descriptive richness of the incident and its specificity to place. Normative data are available, with cut-offs for probable and definite impairment on both sections. The interview has been used in amnesic and demented patients.

The Behavioural Inattention Test (BIT) (Thames Valley Test Company)

The BIT was developed as a standardized test for detecting and measuring the severity of visual neglect, primarily in stroke and head-injured patients. It has been extensively validated, and normative data exist. It consists of six conventional tests, of which the most sensitive is the Star Cancellation Test (see Fig. A1), and nine behavioural tests which use everyday situations to judge visual neglect. Normative data are available, and the battery has now been widely used in stroke patients to assess neglect phenomena.

Six conventional tests:

- Line crossing (Albert's test)
- Letter cancellation
- Star cancellation (see Fig. A1)
- Figure and shape copying
- Line bisection
- Representational drawing

Nine behavioural tests:

- Picture scanning

- Telephone dialling
- Menu reading
- Article reading
- Telling and setting the time
- Coin sorting
- Address and sentence copying
- Map navigation
- Card sorting

The Boston Naming Test (BNT) (Lea and Febiger, Philadelphia)

The BNT consists of 60 line-drawings, graded from very familiar high frequency items such as bed, tree, and pencil through to low frequency items such as trellis, palette, and abacus. Standard stimulus cues (for example, pencil—'used for writing') and phonetic (first-syllable) cues are given if items are unnamed. The test has been widely used in aphasia studies. Limited normative data (which are not IQ adjusted) are available.

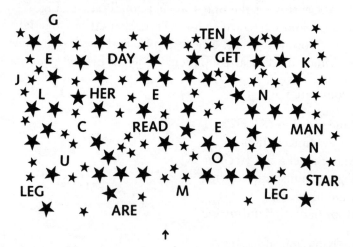

Fig. A1   Star Cancellation Test from the Behavioural Inattention Test (reprinted by permission of Thames Valley Test Company).

Cognitive Estimates Test

In this task, devised by Shallice and Evans, patients are asked to make estimates such as 'What is the largest object normally found in the house?' and 'How fast do racehorses gallop?' The questions cannot be answered directly from general knowledge. They require novel reasoning, and a comparison with information in the individual store of knowledge. Patients with frontal lobe disorders give bizarre answers, when are often not easily modified by asking the patients to reconsider their answers. The specificity and sensitivity of the test have not been well studied, but since there are no good alternative tests it remains clinically useful. A modification of the original test (which contained fifteen questions) is given below. The test is introduced by saying 'I'd like you to make the best guess you can in answer to these questions. Almost certainly you won't know the correct answer, but just make your best guess.' Each answer is scored for unusualness or extremeness. Answers in the correct range score 0. Some responses have to be interpolated, since the scoring system given below cannot cover all possibilities.

Questions and error scores   *Correct range*

1. What is the height of the Post Office Tower?   100–800 feet

>1500	3	<60	3
=1500	2	=60	2
> 800	1	<100	1

2. How fast do racehorses gallop?   15–40 m.p.h.

>50	3	<9	3
=50	2	<15	2
>40	1		

3. What is the best-paid job in Britain today?

Queen/film- or pop-star/ sportsman/ Prime Minister, etc.

manual worker	3
blue-collar worker	2
professionals	1

4. What is the age of the oldest person in Britain today? 104–113

>115	3	<103	3

$= 115$ 2 $= 103$ 1
$= 114$ 1

5. What is the length of an average man's spine?   1'7"–3'11"
   $> 5'0''$ 3 $< 1'6''$ 3
   $> 4'0''$ 2 $= 1'6''$ 2
   $= 4'0''$ 1

6. How tall is the average English woman?   5'3"–5'8"
   $> 6'0''$ 3 $< 5'2''$ 3
   $= 5'11'', 6'0''$ 2 $= 5'2''$ 1
   $= 5'11'', 5'10''$ 1

7. What is the population of Britain?   10–499 million
   > 1000 million   3 < 2 million   3
   > 500 million   2 < 3 million   2
   $= 500$ million   1 < 10 million   1

8. How heavy is a full pint of milk? > 1 lb.–3 lb
   > 3 lb.   3 < 1 lb.   3   (17 oz–43 oz)
   $= 3$ lb.   1 $= 1$ lb.   1

9. What is the largest object normally found in a house?
   $<$ carpet   3   bed, bath, etc.
   carpet   2
   piano, cupboard, sofa   1

10. How many camels are there in Holland?   1–50
    very large number   3
    none   1

Controls obtain mean error score of 4.0 (± 2.0)

Digit span

Digit span is a widely used test of auditory verbal short-term
(working) memory. What it measures is more closely related to the
efficacy of phonological and attentional processes that to what is
commonly thought of as memory (see p. 7). Variations of the task
are included in the Wechsler Memory and Intelligence Scales, in

which the administration and scoring methods used to obtain raw scores and age-scaled scores differ slightly.

In clinical practice the following method is appropriate for determining forward and reverse digit span. For digits forwards, subjects are asked to repeat back progressively lengthening strings of digits in the same order as they are given by the examiner. A practice trial of 2 digits is given, followed by the progressively lengthening strings as shown below. It is important that the digits are read at one per second without clustering. Two different series are given for each string-length. If the subject passes the first or the second, the next length is given. If both are failed, the test is discontinued. The score is the longest series correctly repeated. For reverse digit span, exactly the same method is used, except that the subect is asked to repeat back the digits in reverse order. Again a trial of 2 digits is given initially.

The normal range for digits forwards is 6 ± 1. Even this simple test is affected by age and educational level. Spans of 6 or better are within normal limits; a span of 5 may be marginal or normal, depending on the age and education of the subject; a span of 4 is definitely borderline or impaired; and a span of 3 is always defective. Reverse digit span is 5 ± 1. Hence a reverse span of 3 is borderline or defective, depending upon age and education, and 2 is always defective. In any individual, the difference between forward and backward digit span should not exceed 2.

Digit span is generally vulnerable to focal left hemisphere and frontal lesions. Disorders of attention (for example, delirium or acute confusional states) cause severe reduction, especially in reverse digit span. In Alzheimer's disease, digit span is well maintained initially; but it is reduced in subjects with subcortical dementias.

Digits forwards		Digits backwards	
9—7	2		
4—1	2		
4—8—1	3	6—2	2

6—3—2	3	1—9	2
6—4—3—9	4	2—8—3	3
7—2—8—6	4	4—1—5	3
4—2—7—3—1	5	3—2—7—9	4
7—5—8—3—6	5	4—9—6—8	4
6—1—9—4—7—3	6	1—5—2—8—6	5
3—9—2—4—8—7	6	6—1—8—4—3	5
5—9—1—7—4—2—3	7	5—3—9—4—1—8	6
4—1—7—9—3—8—6	7	7—2—4—8—5—6	6
5—8—1—9—2—6—4—7	8	8—1—2—9—3—6—5	7
3—8—2—9—5—1—7—4	8	4—7—3—9—1—2—8	7
Forward score	__	Backward score	__

The Graded Naming Test (GNT) (NFER–Nelson)

The GNT was designed by McKenna and Warrington to be a stringent test of naming ability, sensitive to mild degrees of anomia. It consists of 30 line-drawings, ranging from low frequency (for example kangaroo, scarecrow, and buoy) to very low frequency (for example, centaur, mitre, and retort). Some examples are shown below (Fig. A.2). Expected scores, based on the WAIS Vocabulary and reading ability, can be calculated. Detailed normative data are available.

Judgement of Line Orientation Test (JLO) (NFER–Nelson)

This task, designed by Benton and colleagues, examines the ability to judge and match angular relationships. The subject views pairs of lines with various orientations, and is required to estimate their angulation with reference to a display of 11 numbered lines spanning 180 degrees, which are viewed simultaneously with the

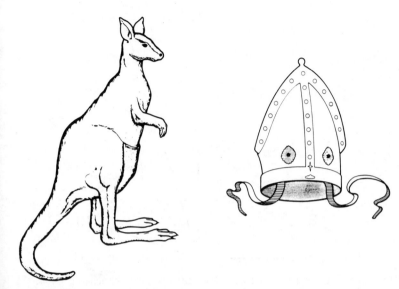

Fig. A2 Graded Naming Test: an example of one of the easier (kangaroo) and one of the harder (mitre) items from the test (reprinted by permission of NFER–Nelson).

target lines (see Fig. A.3). The test consists of 30 trials of increasing difficulty. It is quick and easy to administer, and comes with several parallel forms. Reasonable normative data are available. The test is sensitive to focal right patietal lesions. It is also failed consistently by patients with Alzheimer's disease beyond the earliest stages.

The National Adult Reading Test (NART) (NFER–Nelson)

The NART was developed by Nelson and O'Connell as a quick and simple test to estimate premorbid IQ in patients suspected of suffering from intellectual deterioration. The 50 words constituting the NART are all irregular, in that they cannot be pronounced correctly by applying the usual rules of spelling-to-sound correspondence. For example, the word NAIVE would be pronounced

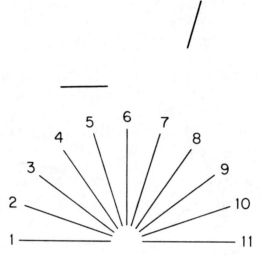

Fig. A3 Judgement of Line Orientation Test (reprinted by permission of NFER–Nelson).

'nave' if one were to decode it phonetically. The principles underlying the test are (i) that the pronunciation of irregular words depends upon pre-existent familiarity with their meaning; and (ii) that reading is a highly overlearnt skill, which is maintained at a high level despite deterioration in other areas of intellectual functioning.

The 50 words of the test are graded in frequency of occurrence in the English language; the initial items (ache, debt, psalm) are familiar to the average adult, while the last words (labile, syncope, prelate) are beyond most people's vocabulary. On the basis of the number of errors produced, a premorbid IQ can be estimated in the range 90–128. For subjects below this range the Schonell Graded Word Reading Test should be used.

While the test remains a valid instrument for estimating premorbid IQ levels in patients with mild dementia, recent research suggests that NART performance declines in moderate Alzheimer's disease. Patients in whom there is a breakdown of the whole-word (lexical) reading route, surface dyslexics, are particularly impaired at reading irregularly spelt words. Their premorbid IQ should be assessed using other measures, such as Raven's Matrices, rather than the NART.

Peabody Picture Vocabulary Test (PPVT) (American Guidance Services Inc., Minnesota, USA) and other word–picture matching tests

The PPVT is an easy-to-administer picture–word matching test consisting of 150 picture plates, each with 4 pictures, arranged in order of difficulty. The subject points to the picture which best fits the word spoken by the examiner. It can also be given in a written-word format. The PPVT was standardized for ages two-and-a-half to eighteen. Hence the early items in the test are extremely easy for the average adult, while the last few are beyond the vocabulary of most people. There is a standard procedure for starting at a level appropriate to the subjects' age and background. From the number of items passed mental-age scores, percentiles, and IQ scores can be derived.

The PPVT remains one of the few standardized tests of single-word comprehension, and as such is useful in patients with suspected semantic comprehension deficits due to focal or progressive degenerative disease, or following a stroke.

Other tests of single-word comprehension, in which the relationship of the target and the distractor pictures has been more systematically varied, have been designed recently. In a semantic memory test battery, we have included a within-category picture-pointing task which is sensitive to comprehension deficits (for example, target: trumpet; array: six musical instruments). The newly-devised PALPA battery (Psycholinguistic Assessment of Language Processing in Aphasia) devised by Kay, Lesser, and Coltheart (publishers, Lawrence Erlbaum, Hove and London) includes a picture-pointing test in which the target is matched with

two semantically-related foils (one closely related and one dis
tantly), one visually-related foil, and one unrelated foil.

Pyramids and Palm Tree Test (Thames Valley Test Company)

This test, recently devised by Howard and Patterson, assesses a
person's ability to access detailed semantic knowledge from word
and from pictures. It can be given in several formats (picture–
picture, word–word, picture–word); but the picture–picture
matching version is perhaps the most useful, since it assesses non
verbal semantic knowledge. There are 52 items in the test. The
subject is presented with three pictures on a single card. One, the
target picture, is displayed below. The subject has to decide which
of the two pictures is most closely associated with the target
Examples include an Egyptian pyramid with a fir tree and a palm
tree (hence the name of the test); spectacles with eye and ear; and
saddle with goat and horse (Fig. A.4). The test remains largely a
research tool, but its usage is likely to increase, since there are few
good alternatives. Normative data are, at present, rather limited
Normal controls make three or fewer errors on the picture–picture
matching version; patients with semantic memory impairmen
make considerably more.

Raven's Progressive and Coloured Progressive Matrices (RPM and RCPM) (NFER–Nelson)

Raven's progressive matrices (RPM) was developed as a 'culture
fair' test of general intellectual inability, although it has subse
quently emerged that educational level has a major effect on
normal subjects' performance. It consists of 60 visually-based
problem-solving tests arranged in blocks of increasing complexity
The initial test items require only pattern matching; the subject is
faced with a large design, part of which is missing; below are six

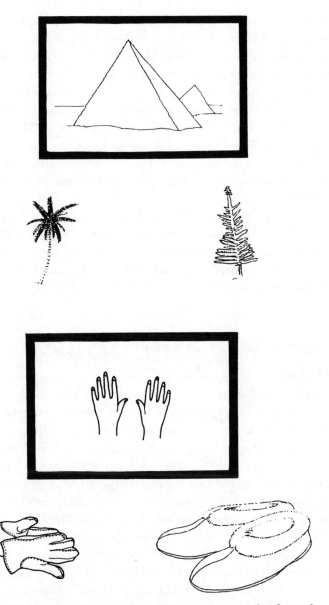

Fig. A4 Pyramids and Palm Trees Test: two examples from the test (reprinted by permission of Thames Valley Test Company).

different small pattern-samples, one of which the subject chooses to complete the larger design above. As the test progresses, the items become more complex, requiring reasoning by analogy rather than simple pattern matching (see Fig. A.5). The test is simple to administer, but takes 45 minutes or so to complete. Detailed normative data with percentile scores are available for ages 8 to 65.

Raven's Coloured Progressive Matrices (RCPM) provides a simplified 36-item format, with norms for children and adults over 65. It also has been used in neuropsychological practice. A greater proportion of the test items are of the pattern matching type than in the RPM.

Both tests are sensitive to brain damage in fairly widely distributed areas, since normal performance depends upon intact visuo-perceptual, attentional, and problem-solving skills. In the absence of visuo-perceptual deficits it is a reasonable test of frontal lobe function.

Recognition Memory Test (RMT) (NFER–Nelson)

This easy-to-administer test of word and face recognition memory devised by Warrington, is becoming widely used in clinical neuropsychological practice. In the face memory part, the subject is shown 50 black and white photographs of unfamiliar male faces. The examiner asks the subject to attend to each for three seconds and to say whether the faces are pleasant or not. After viewing all 50 faces, subjects are then shown pairs of faces, one of which was in the original series. In this forced-choice recognition format, the subjects have to choose which one they have already seen. The word memory part of the test is given with identical instructions. The subject views 50 high frequency words, and then has a two-choice recognition test. Normal subjects perform very well on both parts of the test. Good age- and IQ-standardized normative data are available, including the acceptable range for a discrepancy between word and face recognition. The test is sensitive to episodic

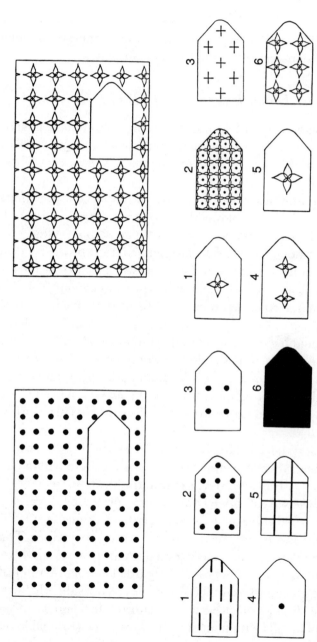

Fig. A5 Raven's Standard Progressive Matrices: examples of two of the easier pattern-matching items from the test (reprinted by permission of the copyright owners, J.C. Raven Ltd.).

memory disorders of all types, and has the advantage of containin verbal and non-verbal tasks in the same format.

Rey Auditory Verbal Learning Test (RAVLT)

This is a verbal serial learning test using 15 common nouns. I provides a measure of immediate recall, evaluates learning ove successive trials, and assesses confabulation and susceptibility t interference.

Five presentations of one list (A) are given, then one presentatio of the second list (B), followed by a sixth recall trial of list A. Th examiner reads list A at one word per second, after givin instructions along these lines: 'I am going to read you a list of words Listen carefully, because when I stop you will have to repeat back a many as you can. It doesn't matter in what order you repeat them.

After the first trial the examiner re-reads the same list a total o five times, using the same instructions, but emphasizing that the subject should include words recalled on previous trials. The orde of the subjects' responses should be recorded each time. After Tria V of list A, the examiner reads list B and asks for recall of this lis only. Finally, following the list B trial, the subject is asked to recal as many words as possible from the original list. This constitute Trial VI.

Recall of Trial I is largely a measure of short-term (working) memory, and, therefore, approximates digit span to within one o two points. It varies according to age and education, so that elderly (>70) subjects recall 5 (± 1) and young professionals recall 7–8 (± 1.5). Normal subjects show considerable learning across Trials I–V, with a mean increment of 5 or 6 words above their Trial I recall, and relatively little age-variation. A drop of 3 or more words between trials V and VI of list A is regarded as abnormal. Further details are given in Lezak's book (see Selected reading below).

Like the RMT, the Rey test is sensitive to episodic memory disorders. Patients with amnesic syndrome show reasonable recall on Trial I, but very little learning over successive trials. They are

lso sensitive to the interference effects of list B, and tend to
onfabulate, producing items extraneous to either list.

ist A	Trials					List B		Trial
	I	II	III	IV	V		Recall	VI
1 Drum	-	-	-	-	-	1 Book	-	-
2 Curtain	-	-	-	-	-	2 Flower	-	-
3 Bell	-	-	-	-	-	3 Train	-	-
4 Coffee	-	-	-	-	-	4 Rug	-	-
5 School	-	-	-	-	-	5 Meadow	-	-
6 Parent	-	-	-	-	-	6 Harp	-	-
7 Moon	-	-	-	-	-	7 Salt	-	-
8 Garden	-	-	-	-	-	8 Finger	-	-
9 Hat	-	-	-	-	-	9 Apple	-	-
0 Farmer	-	-	-	-	-	10 Chimney	-	-
1 Nose	-	-	-	-	-	11 Button	-	-
2 Turkey	-	-	-	-	-	12 Key	-	-
3 Colour	-	-	-	-	-	13 Dog	-	-
4 House	-	-	-	-	-	14 Glass	-	-
5 River	-	-	-	-	-	15 Rattle	-	-
otal	—	—	—	—	—		—	—

Rey–Osterrieth Complex Figure Test

The Complex Figure Test can be used to evaluate both visuo-
constructional ability and visual memory. Subjects are asked to
copy the figure (see Fig. A.6) freehand, without time restriction. A
note should be made of their general approach to the task and
organizational skills. Some examiners use a sequence of different
coloured pencils, which they pass to the subject at 30-second
intervals; but this is probably unnecessary in ordinary clinical
practice. After a delay, typically 30 to 40 minutes, subjects are asked
to reproduce the figure without prior warning. Some neuropsychologists also test recall after a few minutes' delay.

Copying skills are severely disrupted by right hemisphere
damage, often with a tendency to neglect the left side of the figure.
Patients with extensive left hemisphere lesions may also copy the

figure in a disorganized, piecemeal fashion (see p. 141), and fronta patients tend to draw impoverished figures with perseverate elements.

Recall is very poor in patients with the amnesic syndrome, an with selective right temporal lobe damage. Performance on th copy *and* recall portions of the test are extremely poor in patien with moderate to severe Alzheimer's disease; but recall is selectivel impaired in mild disease.

As well as a qualitative assessment, the accuracy of the copie and recalled versions can be scored using the standardized scorin system shown below, which allots a maximum of two points to eac of the 18 elements of the figure.

Normative data	*Copy*	*30-min recall*
Adults <60 yrs.	32±2	22±4
Elderly subjects	28±3	13±4

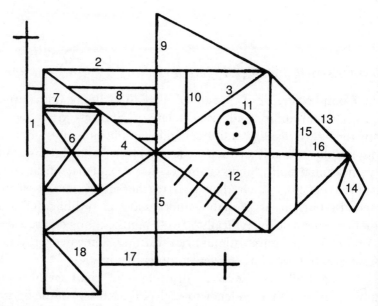

Fig. A6 Rey–Osterrieth Complex Figure Test.

Scoring system

Units	Copy	Recall
1. Cross upper left corner, outside of rectangle		
2. Large rectangle		
3. Diagonal cross		
4. Horizontal midline of 2		
5. Vertical midline		
6. Small rectangle within 2, to the left		
7. Small segment above 6		
8. Small parallel lines within 2, upper left		
9. Triangle above 2, upper right		
10. Small vertical line within 2, below 9		
11. Circle with 3 dots within 2		
12. Five parallel lines within 2 crossing 3, lower right		
13. Sides of triangle attached to 2 on right		
14. Diamond attached to 13		
15. Vertical line within triangle 13, // to right vertical of 2		
16. Horizontal line within 13, continuing 4 to right		
17. Cross attached to low centre		
18. Square attached to 2, lower left		
Total		

Score appears above Copy/Recall columns.

	Placed poorly	Properly placed
Correct	1	2
Distorted or Incomplete	1/2	1
Absent or Not recognizable	0	0 Max.: 36

Rivermead Behavioural Memory Test (RBMT) (Thames Valley Test Company)

The RBMT was developed initially to assess memory recovery i
brain-injured patients. It combines conventional tasks (for ex
ample, orientation and story recall) with more real-life tasks (fo
example, remembering a route and a message) that arguabl
correlate more closely with psychosocial competence. It is an eas
to-use measure, not requiring special professional training t
administer and to score. However, it does take 20 to 30 minutes t
administer. It provides an overall screening score for significan
memory impairment, as well as more detailed scores for each of th
subtests listed below.

1. Remembering a person's first name and surname, tested b
   associating the names with a face (photograph) and asking fo
   the names when the photograph is shown again later (withou
   warning).

2. Remembering ten common objects (which the subject :
   required to name and study), and five faces. The initial stimu
   (objects, faces) are represented with the same number c
   additional distracting objects, and the subject is required t
   identify the objects/faces initially seen.

3. Remembering the gist of a short prose passage, teste
   immediately and again after a twenty-minute delay.

4. Following a route around a room visiting five specified point
   first immediately after being shown and then twenty minute
   later. (A model or drawing can be used for immobile patients.
   The patient is also asked to leave a message (envelope) at on
   point.

5. Remembering to ask for a personal belonging, which is take
   from the patient at the beginning, at the end of the test (20–30
   minute delay).

6. Remembering a particular question (asking about the next appointment), the question being given initially with instructions to ask it when an alarm bell rings twenty minutes later.

7. Ten questions to test orientation in time, place, and person, and one question asking for the date.

Items scored (for RBMT screening score):

1. First name of person in photograph

2. Second name (surname) of person in photograph

3. Remembering hidden belonging

4. Remembering to ask about appointment (question after alarm sounds)

5. Picture (object) recognition (selecting 10 from 20 shown)

6a. Prose recall—immediate (21 ideas)

6b. Prose recall—delayed (20 minutes)

7. Face recognition (recognizing 5 from 10 shown)

8a. Route—immediate (five places)

8b. Route—delayed (about 20 minutes)

9. Route—message (envelope to be left)

10. Orientation

11. Date (correct)

Story recall (logical memory)

A number of different paragraph or story recall tests have been used, all of which derive from the Logical Memory Subtest of the Wechsler Memory Scale (WMS), or are modifications of the Babcock story. In the WMS and WMS-R, two stories are used, each containing 25 elements; the score is taken as the mean of those for the two stories. It is usual to test both immediate recall, and delayed recall after an interval of 30 to 45 minutes. The latter has been shown to be particularly sensitive to episodic memory disorders (for example, the amnesic syndrome, Alzheimer's disease, etc.), and to correlate well with real-life memory difficulties.

The following adaptation can be used:

Mary/Allen/ of North/Oxford/employed/as a cook/in a college,/ reported/at the police/station,/that she had been held up/in Broad Street/that morning/and robbed/of £50. She had three/little children,/the rent was due,/and they had not eaten/for 24 hours./ The Officers,/touched by the woman's story,/made up a purse/for her. Total elements = 24

Subjects should be instructed as follows:

'I am going to read a short story to you now. Listen carefully because when I have finished I am going to ask you to tell me as much of the story as you can remember.' After reading the story, the examiner instructs the patient 'Now tell me everything you can remember.' Recall is again tested after a delay of approximately 30 minutes, without prior warning.

A full credit is given for each element of the story recalled correctly. A half credit is given for synonyms, substitutes, or omissions of an adjective or verb that do not alter the basic idea-unit. The test is very sensitive in normal subjects to the effects of age and general intellectual ability. Table A1 below is a rough guide to the expected normal levels using this test.

Hence, a sixty-year-old of high intelligence would be expected to recall more than 10 elements immediately, and to retain at least 60 per cent after a delay. A normal seventy-year-old of low intellectual ability could recall as little as four elements initially, and retain a third after a delay.

The Token Test

The Token Test is a sensitive and reliable measure of auditory comprehension in aphasic stroke patients, although its value in

Table A1   Age-related norms for the story-recall test

Age	20–39	40–59	60–69	70–79
Immediate recall mean (SD)	10.0(2.5)	8.0(2.5)	7.5(3.0)	6.0(3.0)
Delayed recall as % of immediate mean (SD)	70%(15%)	65%(15%)	60%(20%)	55%(20%)

other language-disordered patients is less clear. It is easy to administer and score, and the material needed can be readily made. Twenty 'tokens' cut from cardboard, plastic, or wood are used. They come in two sizes—big and small; two shapes—circles and squares; and five colours. The original version consisted of 62 commands, graded from the very simple (for example, 'Touch the red circle and touch the small green square') to syntactically complex commands (for example, 'Put the red circle on the green square' and 'Pick up all the squares except the yellow one').

A shortened version, consisting of 36 commands, has been widely used. Educationally standardized normative data are available. For further details see Lezak (under Selected reading below).

Trail Making Test (Halstead–Reitan Test Battery, Reitan Neuropsychology Laboratory, Tucson, Arizona)

This is a quick and easily-administered test of visuo-motor tracking, and of conceptualization and mental 'set-shifting'. It is given in two parts (A and B). Part A consists of a series of circles enclosing numbers from 1 to 25, scattered at random on the page. The subject's task is to join the circles in numerical order as quickly as possible. Part B has both numbers and letters arrayed in the random order. The subject must alternate between numbers and letters: 1 to A to 2 to B to 3 to C, and so on to 13 (see Fig. A.7).

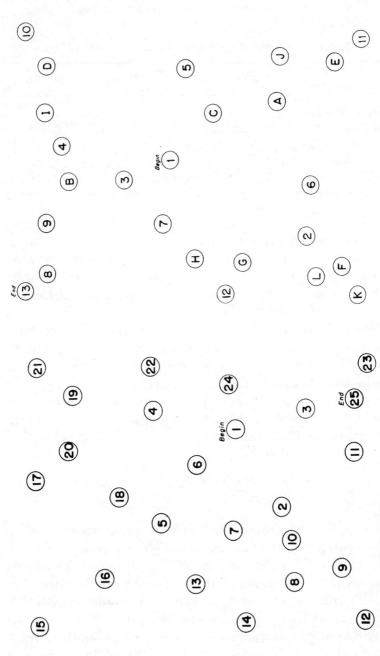

Fig. A7 Trail Making Test parts A (left) and B (right).

Various administration and scoring procedures have been used; but it is usual to point out errors as they occur, to allow self-correction, and to score only in terms of time to complete.

In common with any test which depends upon response-speed, performance on trail making depends markedly on age. Approximate age-adjusted upper limits for normality in seconds are given in Table A2 below:

Table A2   Age-adjusted upper limits for normality (in seconds) on the Trail Making Test

Age	20–39	40–49	50–59	60–69	70–79
Part A	40	45	50	70	100
Part B	90	100	135	170	280

Impaired performance on either part of the test can result from motor slowing, incoordination, visual scanning difficulties, poor motivation, or frontal executive problems. Patients with frontal lobe dysfunction perform disproportionately badly on Part B.

Verbal fluency tests: letter and category fluency

Verbal fluency, sometimes referred to as controlled oral word-association, is a very useful bedside test which is sensitive to frontal 'executive' dysfunction and subtle degrees of semantic memory impairment. A number of versions based on letter and semantic category have been used. The most extensive experience is of 'FAS' for letter fluency, and the category animals.

FAS: Subjects are asked to list as many words as possible beginning with each of the three letters in turn. One minute is allowed per letter. Subjects are told beforehand that proper nouns (personal and place names) and repetitions of words with different suffixes (find, finder, finding, etc.) are not acceptable.

Animals: Subjects are asked to list as many animals as possible in one minute. If this test is given immediately after letter fluency, it i: important to point out that the animal names can begin with any letter.

Scores for the total responses, the number of perseverative errors, and other (intrusive) errors can be obtained. For FAS, it is usual to summate across the three letters. Normal subjects should not perseverate or lose set (i.e. revert to a prior letter). Performance depends on age and education. Young professionals should produce in excess of 45 words for FAS and a total of 30 or below is abnormal. The lowest acceptable total for elderly subjects of low educational attainment is around 25 words. Category fluency is usually superior to letter fluency. For the category animals, normal subjects usually produce 20 exemplars. The lower limit of acceptability ranges from 12 to 15, again depending on age and education.

The Visual Object and Space Perception Battery (VOSP) (Thames Valley Test Company)

This battery of eight visuo-perceptual tests was recently developed validated, and standardized by Warrington and James. Each subset was developed to focus on one component of visual perception, while minimizing the contribution of other cognitive skills. Most of the tasks are based on prior experimental studies performed by the authors. All are sensitive to right hemisphere damage, and normative values are included with the battery.

An initial simple figure–ground discrimination test screens out patients with severe visual handicap. The battery proper consists of four tests of object recognition and four tests of space perception.

Object recognition

1. *Incomplete letters* consists of letters fragmented by varying degrees of masking.

2. *Silhouettes* assesses the subject's ability to recognize common objects photographed from an unusual view.

3. *Object decision* contains arrays of four silhouettes—one real object and three nonsense shapes. The task is to select the real object.

4. *Progressive silhouettes* consists of objects photographed from progressively less rotated viewpoints. The subject is required to identify the object as soon as possible.

Space perception

5. *Dot counting* consists of arrays of five to eight black dots on white cards, which the subject is asked to count.

6. *Position discrimination* consists of two adjacent squares—one has a dot in the centre, and in the other it is off-centre. The subject has to choose the square with the centrally placed dot.

7. *Number location* is similar to the former test, but in this one square contains randomly arranged numbers and the other a single black dot corresponding in position to one of the numbers. The task is to select the number which matches the position of the dot.

8. *Cube analysis* tests the ability of subjects to judge the number of bricks present in a 3-D arrangement of square blocks of increasing complexity.

Wechsler Adult Intelligence Scale (WAIS and WAIS-R) (The Psychological Corporation)

The WAIS and the most recently updated version, the WAIS-R (1981), remain the most widely used test batteries for evaluating general intellectual and neuropsychological ability. For most clinical neuropsychologists, they form the centrepiece of cognitive assessment. A full description of the WAIS is beyond the scope of this book. Its administration and scoring are relatively complex and demand formal training. Interpretation of the results depends upon considerable experience. The subject's behaviour, general approach to testing, and types of errors produced form an important part of the evaluation.

The WAIS consists of 11 subtests (6 verbal and 5 performance), which have been updated in the revised version (WAIS-R). By summating the subtest scores and adjusting for age Verbal, Performance, and Full Scale IQ scores can be derived. An average person should obtain a score of 100 for each, one standard deviation being 15 points. In neuropsychological practice, however, the pattern of individual subtest scores is usually more informative than the overall IQ. Each subtest yields a raw score, which can be converted into a scaled score. An average subject should obtain a scaled score of 10, with the standard deviation being 3 points. But the 'normal' range varies considerably with age; the performance subtests are particularly vulnerable to the effects of ageing. By correcting for age, **age-scaled scores** for each subtest can be derived.

The correlation between specific subtests and individual cognitive functions, and hence pathologies, is relatively poor, because many of the subtests tap several cognitive abilities simultaneously. For instance, Picture Arrangement is dependent upon visuo-perceptual and planning abilities; it is, therefore, susceptible to both right hemisphere and frontal lobe damage.

A full account of the tests and their interpretation can be found in *Neuropsychological assessment* by Lezak (see Selected reading below). A brief description of each of the WAIS-R subtests is included here to aid clinicians with little or no experience of the test battery.

Verbal scales subtests

1. *Information* is a test of general knowledge which consists of 29 questions arranged in order of difficulty from 'How many months are there in a year?' and 'What is a thermometer?' to 'How many Members of Parliament are there in the House of Commons?' and 'Who wrote *Faust*?'

2. *Comprehension* includes 16 open-ended questions which test common sense, judgement, and practical reasoning. Examples

are 'Why do people have to register their marriage?' and 'Why do people who are born deaf have difficulty learning to talk?'

3. *Arithmetic* contains 14 tests of mental arithmetic of increasing complexity, such as 'How much is £4 and £5?' and 'How many hours would it take to walk 24 miles at a rate of 3 miles per hour?'

4. *Similarities* is a test of verbal concept-formation in which the subject must explain what a pair of words has in common. The 14 word-pairs range in difficulty from 'orange/banana' and 'coat/dress' to 'poem/statue' and 'praise/punishment'.

5. *Digit span* tests the ability of subjects to repeat sequences of digits of increasing length first in the same order (digits forward) and then in reverse order (digits backwards). It is also included in the Wechsler Memory Scale. Further details can be found on p. 224.

6. *Vocabulary* consist of 35 words which the subject is asked to define. It starts with extremely common words, such as 'bed' and 'winter', and concludes with the infrequent words 'encumber', 'audacious', and 'tirade'.

Performance scale subtests

Four of the five subtests require motor responses—one writing and three manipulating material. All of them are time-limited, and there are extra credits for rapid completion on several.

1. *Digit symbol* consists of four rows of blank squares each paired with a randomly assigned number from 1 to 9. Above the array is a key which pairs each number with a nonsense symbol. The subject's task is to fill as many blank squares as possible in 90 seconds using the digit–symbol key above.

2. *Picture completion* has 20 incomplete pictures of familiar objects or scenes, with instructions to report which important part is missing. Examples include a knobless door, spectacles without bridge section, and a violin with three pegs.

3. *Block design* is a constructional test in which the subject has to make various patterns using red and white blocks. The subject first copies simple four-block designs made by the examiner, and

then copies increasingly complex designs of up to nine blocks from examples printed on small cards.

4. *Picture arrangement* contains ten sets of cartoon pictures that make up stories. The subject is presented with each set in a scrambled order, and is asked to rearrange them to make the most sensible story in as short a time as possible.

5. *Object assembly* consists of four cut-up jigsaw-like cardboard figures of familiar objects (a manikin, a face in profile, a hand, and an elephant). The subject is presented with each in turn in a scrambled array, and is asked to reassemble the figure as quickly as possible.

Wechsler Memory Scale (WMS) and Wechsler Memory Scale—Revised (WMS-R) (The Psychological Corporation)

The WMS was for many years the standard tool for the assessment of suspected memory disorders. It consisted of six subtests measuring orientation, mental control (attention), digit span, logical memory (story recall), verbal paired associate learning, and visual reproduction of geometrical figures. From these six subtests, a general Memory Quotient (MQ) could be obtained. The MQ was based on the sum of the raw scores. This total raw score was transformed with suitable age-adjustment to the MQ in such a way that it approximated to the Full Scale IQ of the WAIS. Thus an average person should obtain a Full Scale IQ of 100 and an MQ of 100, with the standard deviation of each being 15 points. A discrepancy between IQ and MQ of more than 15 points therefore indicates significant memory impairment. The major criticism of the WMS has been the bias towards verbal memory, the absence of delayed recall conditions for any of the subtests, and inclusion in the MQ score of subtests more dependent upon attentional processes (mental control and orientation) than upon memory *per se*.

The WMS-R is a considerable improvement, and looks set to replace the WMS. It incorporates two new visual memory tests (figural memory and visual paired associates), a new visual counterpart of digit span (visual memory span), a number of administration changes, and most importantly, delayed recall conditions for two of the verbal and two of the visual memory tests. As well as producing raw scores for each of the subtests, separate age-adjusted indices can now be obtained for Verbal, Visual, and General Memory, Attention/Concentration, and Delayed Recall. The memory indices are free from the contaminating effects of attentional deficits. Extensive normative data are accruing, as well as data on patients with common congitive disorders.

The WMS and WMS-R are not appropriate tests for use at the bedside or in the clinic. Their administration requires expertise, and the scoring system is fairly complex. The digit span and logical memory subtests are the most easily adaptable. These provide good measures of attention and of verbal episodic memory, respectively. Everyday versions of these two subtests are described elsewhere (see p. 200 and 215). The remainder of the subtests are described below, to familiarize clinicians with their content, and thus to aid the interpretation of neuropsychological reports.

1. *Information and orientation* contains 14 standard time, place, and person orientation items, plus general information questions (mother's maiden name, President of the USA, etc.).

2. *Mental control* consists of rapid serial counting (20 to 1), alphabet recitation, and serial addition (1, 4, 7, etc.).

3. *Digit span* requires subjects to repeat in forward and reverse order strings of digits of increasing length.

4. *Logical memory* consists of two stories, each of 25 elements, which the subject is asked to recall immediately after hearing and again after a 30-minute delay.

5. *Verbal paired associates* tests subjects' ability to make word-associations. The subject is read a group of 8 word-pairs; half are easy to associate (for example metal–iron, baby–cries) and half

are hard to associate (crush–dark, obey–inch). Subjects are then read the first word of the pair and asked to supply the second word. Up to six trials are given of the same list, but with the word-pairs arranged in different orders. After a delay, the recall is again tested, without prior warning.

6. *Visual memory span* is analogous to digit span, and consists of 'tapping forwards' and 'tapping backwards'. The subject is presented with an array of red squares randomly arranged on a card. On 'tapping forwards', the subject watches the examiner touch red squares in sequences of increasing length, and after each sequence is asked to repeat the sequence from memory. On 'tapping backwards', the subject again watches the examiner touch sequences of increasing length, and is asked to repeat the performance in reverse order.

7. *Visual reproduction* requires the subject to reproduce from memory four geometrical designs, each shown for 10 seconds. After a delay of 30 minutes, the subject is again asked to draw the figures without prior warning.

8. *Figural memory* is a short-term visual memory test in which the subjects look at abstract designs (shaded block drawings) for five seconds, and then, immediately afterwards, are asked to choose from three alternatives which design they have just seen.

9. *Visual paired associates* is analogous to the verbal paired associate test. The subject is shown six abstract line-drawings, each paired with a different colour, and is then shown the drawings alone, and is asked to recall the colour associated with each figure.

The Wisconsin Card Sorting Test (WCST) (NFER–Nelson)

This widely-used test was designed to study 'abstract behaviour' and 'set-shifting ability'. It is sensitive to frontal lobe damage, particularly that involving the left dorsolateral area, and is failed by patients with dementing illnesses, particularly those of subcortical type, but can be impaired in subjects with lesions elsewhere. The subject is given a pack of 64 cards on which are printed one to four symbols (triangle, star, cross, or circle) in one of four colours (see Fig. A.8). The subjects's task is to place them, one by one, under four stimulus cards consisting of: one red triangle, two green circles, three yellow squares, and four blue stars, according to a principle that the patient must deduce from the examiner's responses. For instance, if the principle is colour, the correct placement of the red card is under the red triangle, regardless of form of symbol or number. After 10 correct sorts, the examiner tells the patient to shift. He or she must then work out what is the new sorting dimension. The test begins with colour, then shifts to form, and then to number, then returning again to colour and so on. The most widely used scores are for number of categories achieved (maximum 6) and number of perseverative errors. Perseverative errors occur when the subject continues to sort according to a previously

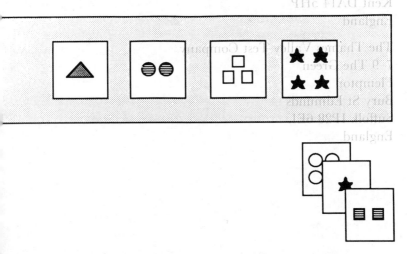

Fig. A8 Wisconsin Card Sorting Test (NFER–Nelson, figure reprinted by permission of Dr Rosaleen McCarthy).

successful principle or, in the first series, when the subj
persists in sorting on the basis of an initial erroneous guess.

The modified card sorting test uses 48 cards and has more expl
instructions for subjects and examiner, but is otherwise fa
similar to the longer version. Further details are given
Neuropsychological assessment by Lezak (see Selected further readin

Addresses of publishers

NFER–Nelson
Windsor
Berks SL4 1BU
England

The Psychological Corporation
Harcourt Brace Jovanovich
High St
Sidcup
Kent DA14 5HP
England

The Thames Valley Test Company
7–9 The Green
Flempton
Bury St Edmunds
Suffolk IP28 6EL
England

Selected further reading

Baddeley, A. D. (1990). *Human memory: theory and practice*. Lawrence Erlbaum, Hove and London.

Benson, D. F. (1979). *Aphasia, alexia, agraphia*. Churchill Livingstone, New York.

Burns, A. and Levy, R. (eds) (1993). *Dementia*. Chapman and Hall, London.

Campbell, R. (ed.) (1992). *Mental lives: case studies in cognition*. Basil Blackwell, Oxford.

Caplan, D. (1987). *Neurolinguistics and linguistic aphasiology: an introduction*. Cambridge University Press, New York.

Code, C. (ed.) (1991). *The characteristics of aphasia*. Lawrence Erlbaum, Hove and London.

Cummings, J. L. (ed.) (1990). *Subcortical dementia*. Oxford University Press.

Cummings, J. L. and Benson, D. F. (1983). *Dementia: a clinical approach*. Butterworth, Boston.

Devinsky, O. (1992). *Behavioral neurology*. Edward Arnold, London.

Ellis, A. W. and Young, A. W. (1988). *Human cognitive neuropsychology*. Lawrence Erlbaum, Hove and London.

Farah, M. (1990). *Visual agnosia: disorders of object recognition and what they tell us about normal vision*. MIT Press, Cambridge, Mass.

Fromkin, V. and Rodman, R. (1988). *An introduction to language*. (4th edn). Holt, Rinehart, and Winston, Fort Worth, Texas.

Heilman, K. M. and Valenstein, E. (1985). *Clinical neuropsychology (2nd edn)*. Oxford University Press, New York.

Hodges, J. R. (1991). *Transient amnesia: clinical and neuropsychological aspects*. W. B. Saunders, London.

Kirshner, H. (1986). *Behavioural neurology*. Churchill Livingstone, Edinburgh.

Lesser, R. (1989). *Linguistic investigation of aphasia*. Edward Arnold, London.

Lezak, M. D. (1983). *Neuropsychological assessment* (2nd edn). Oxford University Press, New York.

Lipowski, Z. T. (1990). *Delirium: acute confusional states.* Oxford University Press.

Lishman, W. A. (1987). *Organic psychiatry: the psychological consequences of cerebral disorder* (2nd edn). Blackwell Scientific, Oxford.

Luria, A. R. (1966). *Higher cortical function in man.* Tavistock, London.

McCarthy, R. A. and Warrington, E. K. (1990). *Cognitive neuropsychology: a clinical introduction.* Academic Press, San Diego.

Margolin, D. I. (ed.) (1992). *Cognitive neuropsychology in clinical practice.* Oxford University Press, New York.

Mesulam, M. M. (ed.) (1985). *Principles of behavioural neurology.* F. A. Davis, Philadelphia.

Parkin, A. (1987). *Memory and amnesia: an introduction.* Basil Blackwell, Oxford.

Schwartz, M. F. (ed.) (1990). *Modular deficits in Alzheimer's-type dementia.* MIT Press, Cambridge, Mass.

Shallice, T. (1990). *From neuropsychology to mental structure.* Cambridge University Press.

Stuss, D. T. and Benson, D. F. (1986). *The frontal lobes.* Raven, New York.

Squire, L. R. (1987). *Memory and brain.* Oxford University Press, New York.

Squire, L. R. and Butters, N. (eds) (1984). *Neuropsychology of memory.* Guildford Press, New York.

Walsh, K. W. (1987). *Neuropsychology: a clinical approach* (2nd edn). Churchill Livingstone, Edinburgh.

Walsh, K. W. (1991). *Understanding brain damage* (2nd edn). Churchill Livingstone, Edinburgh.

Index